The Roots and Fruits of Fasting

Dr. Mary Ruth Swope

The Roots and Fruits of Fasting

Copyright 1998 by Dr. Mary Ruth Swope

Swope Enterprises
P. O. Box 1290
Lone Star, TX 75668

Printed in the United States of America

ISBN: 0-9606936-9-6

CONTENTS

Part 1

The Spiritual Roots and Fruits of Fasting

Part 2

The Evangelistic Potential of Fasting

FOREWORD

At last, millions of Americans are beginning to recognize that we have lost our grip on a powerful spiritual tool used by our biblical forefathers — the discipline of fasting, added to prayer.

Now that many Christians across our nation have begun to recapture the essence of prayer and fasting, our minds are expanding as to its true value — historically, theologically, medically, and in actual practice. The results we are receiving have been dramatic, and I believe they will also be long-lasting.

This easy-to-read, practical book deals with fasting from the spiritual, psychological, and physical points of view. Old and New Testament accounts of fasting are reviewed for us and address the question of why this generation of Christians should obey the scriptural obligation to fast.

We also need to anticipate the physical health benefits of fasting with an understanding of the guidelines for how to engage in a successful fast — short term or long term. These topics, as well as the physiology of fasting, are explained along with the needed wisdom on the symptoms to expect, how to correctly break a fast, and some possible complications.

In addition, suggestions for good nutrition, according to God's plan, are included and complemented with insights on how science and the Bible agree on dietary matters.

I like Dr. Swope's appeal in Part 2 of the book to "fast for the hungry" as a way to create more discretionary income to support Great Commission projects and outreach programs, such as we have here at CBN and at many other ministries.

If you are looking for a practical guide on fasting and prayer, you will enjoy studying this very helpful book — *The Roots and Fruits of Fasting*.

Michael D. Little
President and Chief Operating Officer
The Christian Broadcasting Network

PREFACE

The idea for this book came in an inspired moment
in the middle of the night on March 22, 1998. The
title, the table of contents, and the book jacket were
mine in one hour. Within weeks, the entire project
was ready for the printer.

This was possible because, over the years, I had
compiled extensive information on the subject of
fasting and filed it away in four manila folders. The
availability of this research, taken from library
reading notes, classroom lectures, speeches, religious
magazines, and even two term papers by former
students (one of them dating back to summer 1966),
worked to my advantage.

The major disadvantage, however, is that I cannot
properly credit the original authors for their scientific,
theological, and medical contributions to this book.
In the bibliography I have referenced several books
that were major sources of information for this work.
Without the input from these qualified sources, I
would be left with only my personal testimony about

fasting for these past 22 years. That was not enough for the kind of book I wanted to write.

The major goal of this book is to show how fasting and fitness are synonymous terms whether you are speaking physically, psychologically, or spiritually. Millions of Americans are sick in all three realms, and many are looking for a natural cure for their problems. Extensive scientific evidence shows that fasting, when applied correctly, is a viable treatment for both preventing and reversing a host of physical illnesses common to our society.

In addition, volumes of available books, both modern and historical, present convincing evidence of the value of prayer in changing physical, emotional, mental, and spiritual circumstances. When these two disciplines — fasting and prayer — are applied simultaneously, they provide a total program of calisthenics, discipline, and diet so desperately needed to bring our society back to good health.

Complete directions for how to fast, what to expect from a fast, how to break a fast, and other practical guidelines for fasting can be found in Part 1.

Part 2 introduces readers to the author's special mission: Nutrition With A Mission, Incorporated (formerly known as Kingdom Kalories project) and now called Fast for the Hungry.

This project is designed solely to motivate people to do three things:

- Deny themselves unneeded calories (or other unnecessary items or services).
- Save the money those calories (and other things) would have cost.
- Give the money saved to support philanthropic and/or Great Commission projects and programs.

First tested in 1979, this project has been successful in helping Christians grow spiritually, give abundantly, and improve physically — all at the same time!

It is my dream that this book will make a healthy contribution to these goals.

ACKNOWLEDGMENTS

This book was conceived by my hearing a rhema word from the Lord: "Write Me a book and name it *The Roots and Fruits of Fasting*." Thus, my deepest gratitude for the time, strength, motivation, and ideas goes to the Triune God of the Universe.

My secretary and dearest friend, Charlotte Bates, was my second motivation. To her I owe many debts of gratitude. For two years she has been telling me that many people have phoned our business to ask if I had written a book on fasting. My decision to do so made her very happy.

My new assistant, Diane Daly, has been an incredible help, not only in typing but also in editing and searching various translations of the Scriptures to find precise wording.

I am especially grateful to my only sister, Harriett Krumpelman, who has become my eyes for finding and reading research papers, books, journals, and other resources. She contributed valuable information used in writing this book.

My appreciation also goes to freelance editor, Val Cindric, for adding the finishing touches and to Debra Petrosky for designing the layout of the book. My step-granddaughter, Elise Darbro, played a valuable role in proofing the final manuscript.

Numerous people, authors, former students, a doctor friend, fasting friends, and a secret admirer have influenced the contents of this book.

I am especially grateful to Joel Fuhrman, M.D., whom I have never met, for his book, *Fasting and Eating for Health.* Don't miss getting your own copy; you will develop great confidence in the efficacy of fasting by hearing his testimony.

I send blessings to all of you readers, and especially to those who might be motivated to fast and pray their way to better health.

A Rhema Word

Fasting, like the Lord's supper, like baptism in water, like being born again from above, is an outward expression of an inward condition.

Thus, the form of fasting is not the essential focus of God's moving within and among us.

The essential element of fasting is humility before a Sovereign God who receives our expressions of faith, humility, and obedience as an acceptable sacrifice, born of the urgent desire that God will cause His presence to arise within and among us — so that others are drawn to the Light, Love, and Life of Jesus Christ.

Jack McKinstry
Scottsdale, Arizona
January 1, 1998

Part 1

The Spiritual Roots and Fruits of Fasting

CHAPTER ONE

The Spiritual Roots of Fasting

To make sure we are in agreement, it is important that we understand the meaning of "fasting."

The definition of fasting has not changed throughout history. In the Greek and Hebrew languages, the words for fasting are *nesteuo* and *tsumm.* The Greek word means "to abstain from food or drink"; the Hebrew word means "to cover your mouth."

In our language, fasting means "to abstain from all or certain foods, as in observing a holy day; to eat very little or nothing."[1] Beverages are not mentioned here.

Modern authors and health professionals differ in their definitions. For the purpose of this book, I define fasting as simply the practice of deliberately and willfully denying yourself your usual intake of food and/or drink — mostly for spiritual purposes.

KINDS OF FASTS

1. The normal fast.

This involves no solid or liquid food but only lots of water.

The first account of this kind of fast occurs in Genesis 24:33, which tells us Abraham's oldest and most trusted servant was determined not to eat until he found a wife for Isaac.

Fasting in this way is not a new phenomenon.

2. A total fast.

That means no food and nothing to drink. This kind of fast is for special purposes and must be directed by the Lord.

Scriptural examples include: Moses was 40 days and 40 nights without food or water on the mountain (Exodus 34:28); Paul, after his conversion, spent three days without food or water (Acts 9:9); Esther and all Jews fasted for three days without food or water (Esther 4:16).

This kind of fasting can be dangerous physically and should be undertaken only if God speaks directly to you.

3. The partial fast.

In this fast, certain foods and drinks are eliminated — as when Catholics give up eating meat on Fridays for Lent.

Daniel, for example, refused the king's meat and drink, eating only vegetables and water. Later, he ate "no pleasant food" for 21 days (Daniel 1:12, 10:3). John the Baptist ate only locusts and wild honey, although Scripture does not tell us how long he fasted (Matthew 3:4).

A vegetarian diet would not be an example of a partial fast, in my way of thinking. Vegetarians are not giving up meat for an occasional meal or period of time but, rather, have adopted a vegetarian lifestyle.

A partial fast simply means eating very light meals of fruits or freshly-squeezed juices of fruits or vegetables. Heavy foods — proteins, fats, complex carbohydrates, or grains — are eliminated. Daniel's fast included all the grains but no meat, milk, eggs, or cheese.

Partial fasts include giving up some of our favorite foods, especially those that we crave and tend to overeat.

LIFESTYLES AFFECT FASTING NEEDS

In ancient times, people fasted solely for spiritual reasons. In our day, by contrast, we need to fast both for spiritual and physical (including psychological) renewal and/or development.

Why is this? Let's look at some possible explanations.

1. People in biblical times were eating according to God's dietary laws (Genesis 1:29; Deuteronomy 14; Leviticus 11).

They ate clean meats — mainly lamb and fish — and definitely "no blood." They didn't have processed or man-made foods so their digestive systems were less stressed than ours.

Soda pop and artificially colored, sweetened drinks did not exist. As a result, they had stronger bones. Since there were no salty snack foods or artificial ingredients in their foods, hardening of the arteries and high blood pressure were probably non-existent.

Hamburgers, French fries, doughnuts, and ice cream were unknown foods, as were man-made "fake" foods such as margarine and synthetic eggs. Degenerative diseases caused by a high-fat intake were rare in Bible times.

2. In biblical times, people had a healthier lifestyle.

Physical labor and hard work kept fat from being stored in their bodies. Since their main form of transportation was walking, they enjoyed the many health benefits of daily exercise.

They also went to bed early because they didn't have electric lights, books to read, or televisions to watch. Their stress level undoubtedly was less due to their more relaxed lifestyle.

In addition, they breathed fresh air and drank pure water. That eliminated allergies and constipation problems.

Overall, the way of living in Bible times contributed to better habits and healthier bodies.

The people of Bible times didn't need to fast for physical reasons — as we do today — but they did fast! They fasted regularly two days a week, plus all their commemorative fast days.

For these reasons, I believe our biblical forefathers enjoyed better natural health than we do today. Research and experience also support the benefits of the simple, robust lifestyle they maintained.

My goal is to present fasting as a Christian responsibility and a spiritual discipline that can result in multi-faceted benefits to those who take advantage of it.

FASTING AND REPENTANCE

How do we know that fasting is meant for us in our generation? After all, few Christians are doing it including the clergy!

Fasting is still needed today. Why? Because the heart of man has not changed since Adam and Eve fell from their state of bliss to their sinful state in the garden. A glimpse at America's current spiritual condition provides the evidence.

The church in our modern society cannot be compared in spiritual power with the New Testament Church. Entire denominations today are operating without the power of the Holy Spirit. Women's groups in major denominations are embracing the worship of goddesses of ancient times.

There is little physical healing, few deliverances from demons, and almost no "signs and wonders following" in American congregations. Many church services are devoid of the presence of Jesus. Congregations galore are totally bankrupt of spiritual gifts. They practice a form of religion without any power.

In addition, there is no conviction of sin. In fact, teaching about sin is suppressed. Denominations coddle homosexuals and ordain them as pastors and priests. Church leaders wink at divorce and laugh at the supernatural, choosing to toss aside Jesus' teachings about sin, repentance, heaven, hell, and judgment.

Society's moral failures abound, making us more like Sodom and Gomorrah than we like to admit.

(Remember, God pulverized Sodom and Gomorrah so completely that archeologists, digging for years in search of their ruins, have never found "a hint" of its existence.) I tremble to think how God will judge the church in America as we enter the 21st century.

The time has come for God's people to wake up and for church leaders to call for repentance with fasting and prayer. Why? This short list of our nation's sins screams for a response:

- The killing of 30 million babies without a check of conscience by neither the general public nor most professing Christians.
- The lowering of moral standards that allows fornicators to "run wild" — even in the church.
- The failure of parents and children to learn to live together amicably.
- The destruction of the family unit as a result of "easy divorce."
- Not seriously preventing the drug traffic nor appealing to God for divine protection for our children from the evils of drugs.
- Not adequately protecting the wholesale promotion of statewide gambling lotteries, known to rob and steal from customers as well as entrap them in a gambling addiction.

- Not preventing the removal of prayer from our schools nor the removal of the Ten Commandments from public buildings.
- Permitting the free flow of pornographic materials throughout our stores and the programming of it on television 24 hours a day.
- Our lack of love for one another, especially those of different faiths, colors, and cultures.
- Our failure to study the Word of God and abide by its principles.
- Our lukewarmness toward God in every aspect of our national life.

These symptoms only hint at our decadence. Your lists added to this one would bring a truer picture of why we need to be on our knees before the God of our fathers in repentance — with fasting included.

OUR GREATEST SPIRITUAL WEAPON

The record of the whole Bible indicates that prayer and fasting combined constitute the strongest weapon committed to God's believers. Just as faith needs prayer for its full growth and development, prayer needs fasting for the same reason. Nothing more powerful than prayer and fasting is available to the people of God. It is our greatest, single spiritual weapon.

This being true, it is easy to understand why Satan has and will continue to do everything in his power to keep people from recognizing and using this warfare weapon. The enemy of our souls has blinded our eyes to the truth about fasting and prayer.

The problems we face in America cannot be solved by lawyers, by government officials, by financiers — or by anybody but God's people.

Jesus told His disciples that they were "the salt of the earth." That inferred that they were to give "flavor" to their communities, beginning with their families. In other words, their very presence made the earth acceptable to God. Because of their presence, God was able to continue to deal with the earth in grace and mercy.

Not only does salt flavor, but salt also restrains corruption. So our presence as Christian believers on earth is supposed to slow down corruption in every aspect of human activity — moral, religious, social, and political.

Let me repeat one statement as a way of ending this message. On the basis of the record of the whole Bible, I would say that prayer and fasting combined constitute the strongest single weapon that has been committed to God's believing people. There is nothing more powerful. It is America's spiritual atomic weapon. I trust you will be inspired to join multitudes of us in using this tool from our heavenly Father on a regularly scheduled basis.

OLD TESTAMENT ACCOUNTS OF FASTING

Fasting is a regular practice of people of many faiths — Jewish, Muslim, Hindu, and Seneca Indians, for example. This book, however, will be addressed primarily from the Christian point of view simply because of the author's heritage and experiences.

Let's go first, therefore, to the Holy Bible as our source of information. As in everything, the Bible is the final authority for or against any subject — and fasting is no exception.

The Jewish scribal law required only one compulsory fast — on the Day of Atonement. On that day, the people were to consider it a Sabbath day of rest ". . . in quiet humility; this is a permanent law" (Leviticus 16:31 TLB).

Even young Jewish children were trained to fast on the Day of Atonement as a way of preparing them to obey God as adults and fulfill the requirements of the Law on this national fast day.

There is evidence to show, however, that many Jews also fasted regularly on Monday and Thursday. In addition, they celebrated other times of fasting. In fact, the great revivals spoken of in Scripture were preceded by fasting.

Twenty-three fasting stories are recorded in the Old Testament and 12 in the New Testament. Let's begin with a few examples.

1. Personal fasting for guidance, wisdom, and healing.

The Old Testament first mentions a fast in Genesis 24:33 when Abraham's oldest and most trusted servant was determined not to eat until he found a wife for Isaac.

Concerning Moses, "And he was there with the Lord forty days and forty nights: he did neither eat food nor drink water. And he wrote upon the tablets the words of the covenant, the ten commandments" (Exodus 34:28 KJV).

Later, Moses — while on the mountain receiving the Commandments — did a second forty-day complete fast in an effort to save Aaron and the people from destruction for their sin. (See Deuteronomy 9:18; 10:10.)

Hannah fasted when she wanted a son and was granted a child from God. (See 1 Samuel 1:12-22.)

When King David's little boy was ill, he fasted for seven days and told his servants, "While the child was yet alive, I fasted and wept: for I said, Who can tell whether God will be gracious to me, that the child may live?" (2 Samuel 12:22 KJV). David apparently had experienced or been taught that when circumstances are critical or needs for divine intervention are necessary, fasting and prayer (humiliation) before God are the things to do. God, however, chose not to spare the child, probably because of the circumstances under which the baby was conceived. Still, I doubt that David regretted his efforts to seek divine intervention for the child's healing.

The prophet Daniel received wisdom and understanding about his vision concerning the end times from Gabriel after he confessed his and the nation's sins — and fasted and prayed. (See Daniel 9:3.)

2. Corporate fasting for safety and protection.

In 2 Chronicles 20, we read about King Jehoshaphat who was expecting to be attacked by the Moabites and the Ammonites. Fearing for his life and his nation, he proclaimed a fast throughout all Judah. As a result, the people came out of all the cities of Judah — even wives and children. Why did they come?

- To seek the Lord.
- To unite in declaring God to be their God.
- To fast and pray.

What happened next? The Spirit of the Lord came upon one of the men. Jahaziel prophesied (or predicted) the battle was not theirs, but God's. God spoke through Jahaziel saying:

- You won't need to fight.
- Just stand still and watch God work.
- I'll tell you what to do and how to do it.
- Appoint singers, not soldiers.

When they began to sing and praise God, they won.

Another illustration of corporate fasting and prayer is found in the seventh and eighth chapters of Ezra.

Ezra, a great spiritual leader, asked permission of the king to take a copy of God's laws to Judah and Jerusalem. Since he also wanted to take some gold and silver as an offering to the God of Israel, Ezra gathered about 200 priests and other people to go along. Then he asked the men to fast and pray for three things:

- That they would have a safe trip.
- That they would be protected from bandits.
- That their children would be safe during their absence.

The account says, ". . . that we might afflict ourselves before our God, to seek of him a right way for us" (Ezra 8:21 KJV).

What was the outcome? They were protected and saved from the bandits, and they safely arrived home to Jerusalem.

The Book of Esther gives us a dramatic account of how fasting saved a nation of people from destruction.

An evil government official named Haman concocted a plot to have all Jews killed, including women and children. The massacre was to take place on February 28 of the following year throughout all the provinces of Persia.

When Esther the queen, who was also Jewish, learned of the plot from her cousin, Mordecai, she asked him to gather together all the Jews and fast for her. "Do not eat or drink for three days, night or day." Esther and her maids also fasted.

Then she said, "Though it is strictly forbidden, I will go in to see the king; and if I perish, I perish" (Esther 4:16 TLB). When she did approach the king, he gave her favor and reversed Haman's decree to destroy the Jews.

The Jews chose that day, February 28, to celebrate their victory. Would events have happened this way without fasting and prayer on the part of the people?

3. National fasting for economic restoration.

In Joel chapters one, two, and three, we learn about the terrible conditions of the land at that time in history. All the crops had failed. The cattle were without food and water. There was not even any meat offering or drink offering for the priests.

Joel told them to sanctify a fast. "Who knows?" he said. "Perhaps even yet he will decide to let you alone and give you a blessing instead of his terrible curse. Perhaps he will give you so much that you can offer your grain and wine to the Lord as before! Sound the trumpet in Zion! Call a fast and gather all the people together for a solemn meeting: Bring everyone — the elders, the children and even the babies" (Joel 2:14, 15 TLB).

The responsibility to pray for God's help was given to the spiritual leaders. "The priests, the ministers of God, will stand between the people and the altar weeping; and they will pray, 'Spare your people, O our God; don't let the heathen rule them, for they belong to you'" (Joel 2:17 TLB).

What was the outcome? The Lord did a mighty miracle. Everything was restored. He gave them back the crops that all the locusts had eaten. Once again they had all the food they wanted.

"Praise the Lord, who does these miracles for you. Never again will my people experience disaster such as this.... I alone am the Lord, your God" (Joel 2:26-27 TLB).

4. Fasting and national repentance.

In the Book of Jonah, chapter three, God told the prophet to go to the city of Nineveh and tell them that they were going to be destroyed because of their wickedness. Jonah finally obeyed.

The very day that Jonah entered the city and began to preach that Nineveh would be overthrown in 40 days, the people repented. The king declared a fast whereby everyone put on sackcloth (rough, coarse garments worn at times of mourning).

They cried mightily to God. They said, "Who can tell? Perhaps even yet God will decide to let us live, and will hold back his fierce anger from destroying us" (Jonah 3:9 TLB).

They were right.

"And when God saw that they had put a stop to their evil ways, he abandoned his plan to destroy them, and didn't carry it through" (Jonah 3:10 TLB).

In this account, no one, not even the animals, could eat anything at all or even drink water.

The Old Testament contains 12 other examples of fasting and prayer, illustrating the importance of this practice among the Jewish people.

5. Fasting that pleases God.

God-directed and man-directed fasting is not the same, as the prophet Isaiah's classic presentation in chapter 58, verses 1-12, makes clear.

Men said to God, "We have fasted before you.... Why aren't you impressed? Why don't you see our sacrifices? Why don't you hear our prayers? We have done much penance, and you don't even notice it!"

God quickly gave them the answer for His silence: "Because you are living in evil pleasure even while you are fasting.... What good is a fast when you keep on fighting and quarreling? This kind of fasting will never get you *anywhere* with me" (TLB).

The people had a form of religion and appeared to be godly, but they used their fast days to work on their business bookkeeping, to pay their bills, and have their own way about things. They were not seeking to know God more intimately. They were not wanting to experience more of His power and purpose for their lives.

In these verses from Isaiah 58, God explains that fasting is more than going without food; it is a condition of the heart and is evidenced by the way we treat other people.

- Stop oppressing those who work for you.
- Share your food with the hungry.
- Bring into your homes those who need food.
- Feed the helpless, poor, and destitute.
- Clothe those who are cold.
- Don't hide from your relatives who need help.

What is the result when our hearts are right before God?

- He will shed His own glorious light upon you.
- He will heal you.
- Your godliness will lead you forward.
- Goodness will be a shield before you.
- The glory of the Lord will protect you from behind.
- When you call, the Lord will answer you and quickly reply.

All you need to do is stop oppressing the weak, stop making false accusations, and stop spreading vicious rumors. God says that if you take away the yoke from your midst, the pointing of the finger, and speaking wickedness; if you extend your soul to the hungry and satisfy the afflicted soul, then:

- Your light will shine out from the darkness. The darkness around you shall become as bright as day.
- The Lord will guide you continually and satisfy you with good things and keep you healthy too.
- You will be like a well-watered garden, like an everlasting spring.
- Your sons will rebuild the long deserted ruins of your cities. You will be known as "the people who rebuild their walls and cities."

This is another illustration of God's great generosity in relation to the little He requires of us!

6. When it's too late to fast.
In Jeremiah 14, however, God told Jeremiah:

- Don't pray for these people anymore.
- Don't ask Me to bless them.
- They have not tried to follow My ways.

Then the people told God:

- Yes, we have sinned.
- But help us for the sake of Your reputation.
- We're known as Your people; we carry Your name.
- You are passing through our land. Are You helpless to save us?

But the Lord replied to Jeremiah:

- Don't ask Me anymore to bless them.
- Don't pray for them anymore.
- And when they fast, I will not pay any attention.
- When they bring their offerings and sacrifices, I will not accept them.
- What I will give them in return is war, famine, and disease.

Can a nation wander so far away from God that He will refuse to bless, even if the people fast and pray?

In Jeremiah 36:9, the nation of Israel called another fast, but their circumstances did not change. Why not? God told Jeremiah: "They have not tried to follow Me."

This is a grim thought in light of the condition of our society and the hypocrisy in the church in America today. Dr. D. James Kennedy has this rebuke from God for Christians, "Change your behavior or change your name."

NEW TESTAMENT ACCOUNTS OF FASTING

While there was a lapse of approximately 400 years between the writing of the Old and New Testaments, there was no lapse in the practice of fasting.

In Matthew 6:1-18, Jesus was teaching His disciples regarding three related obligations: the giving of alms, praying, and fasting.

In his book, *Shaping History Through Prayer and Fasting,* author and biblical scholar, Derek Prince (see bibliography), explains that a careful reading of those verses reveals a major emphasis in each case upon the motive of one's action. We are warned against seeking public attention in these matters.

Jesus used the words "*when* you fast," not "*if* you fast." This indicates that the giving of alms, praying, and fasting are expected of all those who follow Christ. (See Matthew 6:16.)

"All disciples" was clarified by the language used in those verses. "When *ye* [plural] pray" (vs. 6), and "when *thou* [singular] prayest" (vs. 7). Derek Prince teaches on the literal translation of these verses (page 78 of his book).

The same situation is true in regard to fasting. "When *ye* [plural] fast" (vs. 16), and "When *thou* [singular] fastest" (vs. 17), clearly teaches that fasting is for every believer.

When Jesus Christ, the Son of God, the Savior of the world, the Coming King who will rule and reign forevermore, says that we should give alms, pray, and fast, I bend my knees and bow my head willing to obey. Why? Because I have learned that He knows how to help me experience the most abundant life possible in the here and now — and for eternity. I am "no fool" to obey what He has recommended or commanded!

1. Jesus fasted.

If we are to pattern our lives after that of our Lord, then we need to learn to fast.

In Luke we read, "Then Jesus, being filled with the Holy Spirit, returned from the Jordan and was led by the Spirit into the wilderness, being tempted for forty days by the devil. And in those days He ate nothing, and afterward, when they had ended, He was hungry" (Luke 4:1-2 NKJV).

2. Jesus expected His disciples to fast.

Christ also made reference to His disciples fasting after He was gone, in response to a question by some Pharisees.

"And Jesus said unto them, 'Can the children of the bridechamber fast, while the bridegroom is with them? As long as they have the bridegroom with them, they cannot fast. But the days will come, when the bridegroom shall be taken away from them, and then shall they fast in those days'" (Mark 2:19-20 KJV).

This is a clear indication to me that our generation should be fasting; these are the days in which the bridegroom has been taken away.

Obedience is the highest form of love.

3. Fasting and the early Church.

The New Testament provides several accounts of individuals who received unusual spiritual insight and personal victory from fasting.

The prophetess Anna "served God with fastings" and was the first person to recognize the baby Jesus as the Child of Promise, the Messiah. (See Luke 2:37-38.)

The disciples of Jesus prayed and fasted before they blessed and sent out many disciples who had been converted at Derbe. Through this the door of faith was opened to the Gentiles. (See Acts 14:23-27.)

Cornelius fasted and received a visitation from an angel to summon Peter. As a result Peter realized that the Gentiles were worthy to be evangelized for Christ. (See Acts 10:30-34.)

Simeon, Barnabas, Lucius, and Manaen fasted, and the Holy Spirit spoke and commissioned Barnabas and Saul to begin the first missionary journey, resulting in the origin of all mission programs. (See Acts 13:1-3.)

Paul and 276 mariners fasted and prayed for 14 days and were spared from losing their lives in a storm at sea. (See Acts 27.)

The apostle Paul is known to have been "in fastings often." Who of us has more to "show and tell" about our Christian life achievements than Paul? (See 2 Corinthians 11:23-27.)

20th CENTURY AMERICA AND FASTING

In 1865, Abraham Lincoln called for a day of National Humiliation — a day of fasting and prayer. In the proclamation he wrote for this occasion, he acknowledged that the people, including the government, had forgotten ". . . the hand which preserved us in peace."

"We have become too self-sufficient to feel the necessity of redeeming and preserving grace," Lincoln wrote, "too proud to pray to the God who made us. It behooves us, then, to humble ourselves before the offended Power, to confess our national sins, and to pray for clemency and forgiveness."[2]

This sounds like the Old Testament kings and priests when they called for a national fast.

At the turn of the 20th century, there was a definite shift in attitude about fasting. Schools of theology no longer included it in their curriculum. The social gospel was in its infancy and soon infamous to the pentecostals and evangelicals who, in part, remained true to the fasting message.

Today, few American Christians have either knowledge of or experience in fasting. One major reason for this is that neither our theological or medical "giants" believe in or practice fasting themselves. Few pastors will permit the subject to be taught in their churches. I know from personal experience that most church leaders and medical doctors do not want to deal with the subject.

It is possible, however, to find many examples of individuals who have lived fasted lives. My personal observation of these people is that they could be called the giants of the Christian faith. Their records of achievements for the kingdom of God are indisputably among the very best.

In my experience, Catholics more than Protestants have embraced the doctrine of fasting. Denying themselves foods and/or meals around the season of Lent and other times are well known.

For years Muslims have fasted at Ramadan from dawn till dusk and even deny themselves bathing, the wearing of perfumes, smoking, drinking, and other indulgences.

The present-day call to America to fast, pray, and seek God's face was initiated by Dr. Bill Bright of

Campus Crusade for Christ. He felt called by God to ask Americans to prepare themselves personally, as a church, and as a nation for a spiritual revival so that the Great Commission could be fulfilled.

At Dr. Bright's first three-day meeting of Christian leaders in 1994, Dr. Adrian Rogers said, "I believe as the West goes, so goes the world. And as America goes, so goes the West. And as the Church goes, so goes America. And as believers fast and pray, so goes the Church."[3]

This event led to an annual three-day fasting and prayer conference — first in Los Angeles (1995), then in St. Louis (1996), Dallas-Fort Worth (1997), and in Houston, Texas (1998).

The prayer and fasting idea has become a national (even international) movement. It is estimated that from March 1 to April 9, 1998 as many as one million Americans attempted a 40-day fast.

Will God hold back His hand of judgment against morally decadent America because of this fasting effort?

If recorded history is any indication, it is hopeful that He will. There is always one example before us, however, to show that we cannot be sure. He did not spare the people of Judah in the time of Jeremiah.

With a quote from Jeremiah 15:1-7, I close this chapter:

Then the Lord said to me, "Even if Moses and Samuel stood before me pleading for these people, even then I wouldn't help them — away with them! Get them out of my sight! And if they say to you, But where can we go? Tell them the Lord says: Those who are destined for death, to death; those who must die by the sword, to the sword; those doomed to starvation, to famine; and those for captivity, to captivity. I will appoint over them four kinds of destroyers, says the Lord — the sword to kill, the dogs to tear, and the vultures and wild animals to finish up what's left. Because of the wicked things that Manasseh, son of Hezekiah, king of Judah, did in Jerusalem, I will punish you so severely that your fate will horrify the peoples of the world.

Who will feel sorry for you, Jerusalem? Who will weep for you? Who will even bother to ask how you are? You have forsaken me, and turned your backs upon me. Therefore I will clench my fists against you to destroy you. I am tired of always giving you another chance. I will sift you at the gates of your cities and take from you all that you hold dear, and I will destroy my own people because they refuse to turn back to me from all their evil ways (TLB).

SHOULD THIS GENERATION FAST?

It goes without saying that America is in the middle of a moral free-fall. Our leaders in government and all other fields of endeavor are a reflection of the immorality taught in school textbooks and displayed on television, in movies, rock music, theater productions, magazines, etc.

Public school curriculum includes instruction on many demonically inspired subjects. The teaching of explicit sex materials has produced a sexually active new culture with many students having a dozen or more sex partners before they graduate from high school.

It is frightening to see how many Americans are satisfied at seeing the Ten Commandments taken down from courtroom and school building walls and who apathetically allow manger scenes to disappear from public places at Christmas time.

Economic disaster looms ominously over our nation as Americans refuse to balance their personal, corporate, or national budgets. Rome didn't either. The same economic fate that has befallen Argentina, Mexico, and several Far East countries awaits our nation unless God intervenes.

More and more the United Nations flag is appearing in our public buildings, over military bases, and many other places. Is our republic being challenged?

These events are not even the tip of the iceberg! If the whole truth about our decadence was revealed at one time, millions of us would be shaken to the core. We would be crying out to God from the depths of our souls.

We should fast for a thousand reasons. One of them is that we, as evangelical Christians, will soon be a despised and oppressed minority!

Already movies and television shows portray Christians as bigots, censors, intolerant, narrow-minded, idiots, and charlatans. This caricature is a real threat to freedom and our present lifestyle.

The traditional family is disappearing and being replaced by "newer forms" of family structure. The undermining of this backbone of our culture and the richest source of American heritage has cut the fabric of our nation to shreds.

Violence is becoming normal behavior. The daily news chronicles those who have been robbed, beaten, raped, gun-downed, and left for dead.

These are but a few examples of why I believe it is time for American Christians to seek God's face, to weep, to repent, and to fast and pray. The precedent for such action is fully supported from the Scriptures.

WHY CHRISTIANS SHOULD FAST

The work of George Wingate of Florida outlines the biblical reasons Christians should fast. (It was not possible to locate Mr. Wingate to give him proper credit for his work, nor to secure the exact Bible translations referenced. Nonetheless, he shall someday receive his reward.)

1. In obedience to God's Word.

Isaiah 58:6-9: "Is not this the kind of fast I have chosen: to loose the chains of injustice and untie the cords of the yoke, to set the oppressed free and break every yoke?

"Is it not to share your food with the hungry and to provide the poor wanderer with shelter — when you see the naked, to clothe him, and not to turn away from your own flesh and blood?

"Then your light will break forth like the dawn, and your healing will quickly appear; then your righteousness will go before you, and the glory of the Lord will be your rear guard.

"Then you will call, and the Lord will answer; you will cry for help, and He will say: Here am I."

Joel 2:12: "'Even now,' declares the Lord, 'return to me with all your heart, with fasting and weeping and mourning.'"

Matthew 17:21: "But this kind of demon does not go out except by prayer and fasting."

Matthew 9:15: "Jesus answered, 'How can the guests of the bridegroom mourn while he is with them? The time will come when the bridegroom will be taken from them; then they will fast.'"

2. To be humbled in order to receive the grace and power of God.

James 4:10: "Humble yourselves before the Lord, and He will lift you up."

Philippians 2:8: "And being found in appearance as a man, He humbled Himself and became obedient to death, even death on a cross!"

Psalm 35:13: "Yet when they were ill, I put on sackcloth and humbled myself with fasting."

1 Peter 5:5-6: "Young men, in the same way be submissive to those who are older. All of you, clothe yourselves with humility toward one another, because God opposes the proud but gives grace to the humble. Humble yourselves, therefore, under God's mighty hand, that He may lift you up in due time."

Deuteronomy 9:3-4: "But be assured today that the Lord your God is the one who goes across ahead of you like a devouring fire. He will destroy them; He will subdue them before you. And you will drive them out and annihilate them quickly, as the Lord has promised you.

"After the Lord your God has driven them out before you, do not say to yourself, 'The Lord has brought me here to take possession of this land because of my righteousness.' No, it is on account of the wickedness of these nations that the Lord is going to drive them out before you."

Ezra 8:21: "There, by the Ahava Canal, I proclaimed a fast, so that we might humble ourselves before God and ask Him for a safe journey for us and our children, with all our possessions."

2 Chronicles 7:14: "If my people, who are called by my name, will humble themselves and pray and seek my face and turn from their wicked ways, then will I hear from heaven and will forgive their sin and will heal their land."

3. To overcome temptations in the areas that keep one from moving in God's power.

Luke 4:1-2: "Jesus, full of the Holy Spirit, returned from the Jordan and was led by the Spirit in the desert, where for forty days He was tempted by the devil. He ate nothing during those days, and at the end of them He was hungry."

Luke 4:14: "Jesus returned to Galilee in the power of the Spirit, and news about Him spread through the whole countryside."

4. To be purified from sin. (Either from your sins or the sins of others.)

Daniel 9:3: "So I turned to the Lord God and pleaded with Him in prayer and petition, in fasting, and in sackcloth and ashes."

1 Samuel 7:6: "When they had assembled at Mizpah, they drew water and poured it out before the Lord. On that day they fasted and there they confessed, 'We have sinned against the Lord.' And Samuel was leader of Israel at Mizpah."

Nehemiah 9:1-2: "On the twenty-fourth day of the same month, the Israelites gathered together, fasting and wearing sackcloth, and had dust on their heads. Those of Israelite descent had separated themselves from all foreigners. They stood in their places and confessed their sins and the wickedness of their fathers."

Jonah 3:5: "The Ninevites believed God. They declared a fast, and all of them, from the greatest to the least, put on sackcloth."

5. To become weak, so God's power can be strong.

Psalm 109:24: "My knees give way from fasting; my body is thin and gaunt."

2 Corinthians 12:9-10: "But He said to me, 'My grace is sufficient for you, for my power is made perfect in weakness.' Therefore I will boast all the more gladly about my weaknesses, so that Christ's power may rest on me. That is why, for Christ's sake, I delight in weaknesses, in insults, in hardships, in persecutions, in difficulties. For when I am weak, then I am strong."

6. To obtain God's support in order to accomplish His will.

Acts 13:3: "So after they had fasted and prayed, they placed their hands on them and sent them off."

Acts 14:23: "Paul and Barnabas appointed elders for them in each church and, with prayer and fasting, committed them to the Lord, in whom they had put their trust."

7. When asking for God's help in a difficult situation.

1 Samuel 12:16: "Now then, stand still and see this great thing the Lord is about to do before your eyes!"

Esther 4:16: "Go, gather together all Jews who are in Susa, and fast for me. Do not eat or drink for three days, night or day. I and my maids will fast as you do. When this is done, I will go to the King, even though it is against the law. And if I perish, I perish."

Matthew 17:21: "But this kind does not go out except by prayer and fasting."

Isaiah 58:6: "Is not this the kind of fasting I have chosen: to loose the chains of injustice and untie the cords of the yoke, to set the oppressed free and break every yoke?"

8. For help in seeking God's direction.

Ezra 8:21: "There, by the Ahava Canal, I proclaimed a fast, so that we might humble ourselves before our God and ask him for a safe journey for us and our children, with all our possessions."

Ezra 8:23: "So we fasted and petitioned our God about this, and He answered our prayer."

9. To provide understanding when extensively studying the Bible or seeking divine revelation.

Jeremiah 36:9: "In the ninth month of the fifth year of Jehoiakim, son of Josiah, king of Judah, a time of fasting before the Lord was proclaimed for all the people in Jerusalem and those who had come from the towns of Judah."

Daniel 9:2-3: ". . . in the first year of his [King Darius'] reign, I, Daniel, understood by the books the number of years specified by the word of the Lord, given through Jeremiah the prophet, that He would accomplish seventy years in the desolation of Jerusalem. Then I set my face toward the Lord God to make request by prayer and supplications, with fasting, sackcloth, and ashes."

Daniel 9:22-23: "And he informed me, and talked with me, and said, 'O Daniel, I have now come forth to give you skill to understand. At the beginning of your supplications the command went out, and I have come to tell you, for you are greatly beloved; therefore consider the matter, and understand this vision . . .'"

Other Scriptural reasons for fasting would include the following:

1. In times of need for special power to overcome Satan.

"'However, this kind does not go out except by prayer and fasting'" (Matthew 17:21 NKJV).

2. In times of special need for the work of God and in times of persecution and opposition toward the people and work of God.

". . . in stripes, in imprisonments, in tumults, in labors, in sleeplessness, in fastings;" (2 Corinthians 6:5 NKJV).

". . . in weariness and toil, in sleeplessness often, in hunger and thirst, in fastings often, in cold and nakedness" (2 Corinthians 11:27 NKJV).

3. In times of exceptionally earnest prayer, whatever your prayer may concern.

"Do not deprive one another except with consent for a time, that you may give yourselves to fasting and prayer; and come together again so that Satan does not tempt you because of your lack of self-control" (1 Corinthians 7:5 NKJV).

4. In times of need for special guidance concerning the work of God and for power and blessings upon those the

Lord leads us to send out from our midst as mission-aries.

"Then having fasted and prayed, and laid hands on them, they sent them away" (Acts 13:3 NKJV).

5. In times of special worship and communion with and enjoyment of the Lord.

"So Moses went into the midst of the cloud and went up into the mountain. And Moses was on the mountain forty days and forty nights" (Exodus 24:18 NKJV).

"So he was there with the Lord forty days and forty nights; he neither ate bread nor drank water. And He wrote on the tablets the words of the covenant, the Ten Commandments" (Exodus 34:28 NKJV).

"When I went up into the mountain to receive the tablets of stone, the tablets of the covenant which the Lord made with you, then I stayed on the mountain forty days and forty nights. I neither ate bread nor drank water (Deuteronomy 9:9 NKJV).

"And I fell down before the Lord, as at the first, forty days and forty nights; I neither ate bread nor drank water, because of all your sin which you committed in doing wickedly in the sight of the Lord, to provoke Him to anger (Deuteronomy 9:18 NKJV).

6. Praying through a personal crisis.

In a time of severe crisis, David sought God for the life of his child. As the child lay dying, David fasted and prayed.

"David therefore besought God for the child; and David fasted, and went in, and lay all night upon the earth" (2 Samuel 12:16 KJV).

When the crisis was past, David renewed his normal routine, although the prayer of his heart went unanswered and the child died. Remember, therefore, that fasting never guarantees the answer you seek in prayer. In fact, fasting will cause you to seek God's will, whatever the answer may be.

7. Seeking the perfect will of God.

Ezra, the priest, sought the Lord's leading in order to be found directly in the center of His will.

"Then I proclaimed a fast there, at the river of Ahava, that we might afflict ourselves before our God, to seek of him a right way for us, and for our little ones, and for all our substance" (Ezra 8:21 KJV).

Appetites are so distracting! They interfere with our prayer life, our quiet time, and our overall spirituality. Fasting removes them and gives us time — that fleeting commodity — to address Deity with the petitions of our prayer. We have more time to listen, to learn, and to lean upon the Lord when fasting is a factor in our walk.

8. Fasting is a Christlike self-denial.

The rich young ruler discovered that self-denial and discipleship go hand-in-hand (Matthew 19:16-23).

The body that is preoccupied with appetite cannot be occupied with the Lord, the needy, and the lost. Self-denial afflicts the soul and disciplines the body so that the priorities of God come sharply into focus. Once in focus, they impact the heart and change our perspective and our behavior.

9. Fasting brings healing.

Healing takes many forms. We speak here of both spiritual and physical well-being.

"Then shall thy light break forth as the morning, and thine health shall spring forth speedily: and thy righteousness shall go before thee; the glory of the Lord shall be thy reward" (Isaiah 58:8 KJV).

Although we will give this passage further treatment later, please be aware that the Bible endorses fasting for one's physical health.

Moreover, consider the spiritual condition of a young lad whose story appears in the book of Matthew. The disciples made every attempt to exorcise the demon but experienced futility. Jesus told them they lacked faith on the one hand, and they lacked fasting on the other: "Howbeit this kind goeth not out but by prayer and fasting" (Matthew 17:21 KJV).

Healing in any form, therefore, can be affected by the practice of fasting. Both the physical and spiritual aspects of the fast promote one's overall health.

10. Self-abnegation brings us closer to God.
A still, small voice eludes us when the roar of self rages and wails. Silence the rampage, and the voice of God seems more distinct and conspicuous. Control the passion, the lust, and the egocentricity that usually compels us, and the Lord may find an opportunity to speak more clearly and incline His ear to our prayer.

Scripture does not limit such access to God to the Old Testament era. Fasting will demonstrate to us that the Lord will intervene today when we approach Him in this way.

(The following three lists are taken from page 724 of *Dake's Annotated Reference Bible*[4] in relation to Isaiah 58. I am grateful to the Dake family for their permission to share this information with readers.)

WHAT DOES NOT CONSTITUTE A FAST?

- Practices about which we complain.
- Afflicting the soul to attract God.
- Doing pleasures.
- Exacting all labors.

- Contention and debates.
- Smiting with the fist of wickedness.
- Making voice to be heard in public.
- Bowing the head like a bulrush to make an impression on others.
- Spreading sackcloth as ashes under us.
- Having a sad countenance, disfiguring the face, and making a show to be seen of men (in fasting or any other practice, Matthew 6:16-18).

WHAT DOES CONSTITUTE A FAST?

- To loose the bands of wickedness.
- Undo the heavy burdens.
- Let the oppressed go free.
- Break every yoke.
- Deal bread to the hungry.
- Shelter the cast out.
- Cover the naked.
- Not covering up your own faults.
- To call upon and cry to God.
- Cease accusing others.
- Stop speaking vanity.
- Having compassion on the hungry.
- To satisfy the afflicted soul.
- Keep from desecrating Sabbaths.
- Abstain from doing own pleasure on Sabbaths.
- Love and delight in Sabbaths.

- Call the Sabbaths holy to the Lord.
- Call the Sabbaths honorable.
- Honor God in all things.
- Live an unselfish life.
- Live for God and not for your own pleasure
- Speak God's word, not your own.
- Abstain from food.

TWENTY BLESSINGS FROM A FAST

- Then you shall have light as day.
- Your health will spring forth speedily.
- Your righteousness will go before you.
- God's glory will be your rear guard.
- Then you will call and receive answers to prayer.
- You will cry and God will answer you.
- Then your light will rise in obscurity.
- Your darkness will be as the noon day.
- The Lord will guide you continually.
- He will satisfy you in drought.
- He will make your bones fat.
- You will be like a watered garden.
- You will be like an unfailing spring of water.
- Your waste places will be built.
- You will raise up the foundations of many generations.
- You will be called "the repairer of the breach" and "the restorer of paths to dwell in."

- Then you will delight yourself in the Lord.
- I will cause you to ride upon the high places of the earth.
- I will feed you with the heritage of Jacob your father, for I have spoken it from My mouth.

QUESTIONS AND ANSWERS

When is it wise to fast?

- When we purpose to seek a closer walk with God.
- When we need to humble ourselves before God.
- When we face humanly impossible situations.
- When we need God's guidance.
- When we need healing (Isaiah 58:8).

What results can you expect?

". . . and your Father who sees in secret will reward you openly" (Matthew 6:18 NKJV).

Believe it! Please believe it, and keep reading for more specific results we can expect from the discipline of fasting.

CHAPTER TWO

The Fruits of Fasting

Our fasting is only a continuation of a pattern that began with the history of the Jewish people. They fasted regularly — two days a week.

From the time of Moses forward, fasting was an accepted practice for believers. The Pharisees and the disciples of John the Baptist fasted; the practice can be traced down through the generations until today.

In Mark 2:18-20, Jesus gives a simple parable about a bridegroom.

- The bridegroom was Jesus Himself.
- The children of the bride chamber were the disciples. While the bridegroom was with them, they didn't need to fast (when Christ was on earth).

- When the bridegroom was taken away (while Christ is in heaven before He returns to earth again), the disciples were expected to fast.

In Matthew 6:1-18, Jesus talks with His disciples on three related duties — giving alms, praying, and fasting. These three duties have not been rescinded!

We need to ask ourselves two questions:

1. What would God like for me to do about all I am learning about fasting?

2. Once I know God's will for my role in the end times, am I willing to commit myself to doing God's will, even if it means moving out of my present comfort zone by fasting?

"He who will not change fears not his God" (Psalm 55:19).

Are we willing to make some changes in our lives? Do we really respect and fear the Lord?

Each of us must decide for ourselves.

FRUITS THAT ACCRUE TO THE SPIRIT

There are rewards of fasting that accrue to the spirit, the soul, and the body. God in His wisdom has provided a reward for every part of His crowning creation, the human being.

Let's look at the spiritual rewards of fasting.

1. Fasting provides the ideal milieu for getting closer to God in our relationship with Him.
Somehow our spiritual receptor sites get cleaned out, and we are able to hear His still small voice more clearly.

Acts 13:2-3 says, "As they ministered to the Lord and fasted, the Holy Spirit said . . ." (NKJV). Fasting helped open the ears of early believers to the voice of God for service.

Derek Prince said it so well in a taped sermon, "It is never easier to hear God speak to us than in a time of fasting and praying."

That has been my own experience. In fact, that is one of my main reasons to fast one day a week. I need to hear from God about life's affairs and events. Humbling myself in fasting helps with this.

2. Fasting increases spiritual brokenness.
Dick Eastman of Every Home for Christ of Colorado Springs, Colorado gave another spiritual fruit of fasting when he wrote, "Fasting increases spiritual brokenness."[5]

Psalm 69:10 says, "I have broken my spirit with fasting" (NEB).

There are many words in the dictionary to describe "broken." The one that applies here is "to be weakened or beaten — a broken spirit." That describes what happens to the spirit when food is withheld; it is weakened, and then it yields to the heavenly pull.

3. Fasting increases our spiritual control.
Psalm 35:13 says, "I mortified [put to death] myself [my flesh] with fasting" (NEB).
Paul spoke of the fruit of the Spirit as including temperance (self-control). Fasting helps produce this fruit.

4. Fasting helps us prevail in prayer with God.
"So we fasted and besought our God for this: and he was intreated of us" (Ezra 8:23 KJV).
When we are willing to set aside the appetite of the body to concentrate on prayer, it demonstrates that we mean business with God.

5. Fasting with prayer may bring mercy from God rather than judgment.
". . . Turn to Me with all your heart, with fasting, with weeping . . . For He is gracious and merciful" (Joel 2:12-13 NKJV).

6. Fasting may reveal to us the will of God for our lives.
Simon Peter's experience with Cornelius in Acts 10:30-36 is an illustration of this. God showed Peter that he was to take the gospel to the Gentiles — something that had been forbidden by Jewish law.

7. Fasting increases spiritual power over Satan.

"Then Jesus, being filled with the Holy Spirit . . . was led by the Spirit into the wilderness, being tempted for forty days . . . He ate nothing.... Now when the devil had ended every temptation, he departed from Him.... Then Jesus returned in the power of the Spirit to Galilee" (Luke 4:1-2, 13-14 NKJV).

The outflow of Christ's power came after His time of fasting.

An interesting point here is that Jesus did not move into formal ministry, did not heal or deliver the people from demons, until after his 40-day fast.

In the time of John Wesley here in America, no person was permitted to be a pastor in the Methodist Church until he had fasted for 40 days.

These examples illustrate the reality of the statement: Fasting increases spiritual power.

8. Fasting increases spiritual usefulness.

"Now there was one, Anna, a prophetess . . . a widow of about eighty-four years, who did not depart from the temple, but served God with fastings and prayers night and day" (Luke 2:36-37 NKJV).

If fasting aids our spirit in hearing His voice, then it also increases our usefulness to God, assuming we are obedient to what He has spoken. Are you willing to serve God with ongoing fasting? If done for the

right reasons, it will make a big difference in your life
— for certain.

FRUITS THAT ACCRUE TO THE SOUL

What is the soul? It is man's intellect, emotions,
and will.

Fasting is a spiritual discipline of the body that
humbles the soul. David wrote, "I humbled myself
with fasting" (Psalm 35:13 NKJV).

A dictionary definition of *humble* is "to lower in
pride, make modest or humble in mind. To lower in
rank, condition or position; to abase."[6]

Every bit of that has happened to me as I withheld
food from my body, especially on extended fasts of
seven days and longer.

1. Fasting disciplines the soul and its appetites.

Fasting afflicts the soul according to Isaiah 58:3 and
Leviticus 16:31. That means it disciplines our minds,
emotions, and will; it causes the soul pain and suffering, distress and to be overthrown.[7]

How so, you ask?

Fasting appears to modulate excessive human
appetites such as food, drink, excessive sensual desires,
egocentricity, etc.

Paul wrote plainly about this in 1 Corinthians 6:12-
13, ". . . if I think they might get such a grip on me

that I can't easily stop when I want to. For instance, take the matter of eating. God has given us an appetite for food and stomachs to digest it. But that doesn't mean we should eat more than we need. Don't think of eating as important, because some day God will do away with both stomachs and food" (TLB).

My own experience is that fasting has taken away my cravings and stopped my binging on food.

Fasting helps us prevail in prayer over these matters. All of these represent fruits, benefits, or rewards to the soul of man.

2. Fasting opens our spiritual ears.

When the fast is done for the right reason (as unto the Lord), the spirit gets stronger while the body "simmers down a bit" — in some ways weakens. The Holy Spirit can get His messages through easier, and that always brings renewed strength, peace, joy, and contentment.

3. Fasting refreshes and strengthens our spiritual man.

The Holy Spirit almost always gives us new insights into our thinking, believing, and behavior patterns. If we are obedient to His revelations, we come off a fast spiritually refreshed and stronger in purpose and motivation.

4. Fasting helps to produce the fruit of self-control, the control of one's emotions, desires, actions, etc.

The will is the component of our soul that makes decisions to do or not to do, to say or not to say, to act or not to act. Strengthening the spirit by fasting yields better self-control. (See Galatians 5:22-25; Colossians 3:12.)

5. Fasting helps us submit to God's will.

In fasting with prayer, God empowers our soul to will and to do His good pleasure. (See Philippians 2:13.) It is our choice everyday to do what God wants us to do or what our flesh and soul want us to do. The powerful tool of fasting makes us willing to submit our will to God each day. Permitting God to have His will in our lives is, of course, a main purpose in living.

6. Fasting helps us focus on Jesus.

The fruits of fasting also have an effect on the mind — our wisdom, knowledge, and reasoning areas. The mind is the battlefield of our lives. It must be constantly renewed by the Word of God or it will be an unruly member.

We must bring our thoughts into captivity and produce within us "the mind of Christ" (2 Corinthians 10:5).

"For consider Him . . . lest you become weary and discouraged in your souls" (Hebrews 12:3 NKJV). When we fast, we have great opportunity to "look unto Jesus" and always become victorious in our thoughts.

7. Fasting produces the fruit of the Spirit in our lives.
Fasting for the purpose of seeking a closer relationship with God will definitely produce the fruit of the Holy Spirit in the person fasting — hopefully a major goal of every believer!

FRUITS OF FASTING FOR THE BODY

One of the greatest physical benefits of fasting is that your spirit gets strong enough to dictate to your flesh what it will or will not permit. Left to its own desires, the flesh becomes unrestrained in its wants; it will do almost anything to have its way.

Fasting, with prayer, breaks that power. It is from this strength that a person often gives up addictions during a fasting time. Food is one area of our lives where human, unrestrained appetites do great damage — physically, psychologically, financially, and spiritually.

Other physical benefits of fasting are numerous. Here is a lengthy list:

1. Our taste buds get renewed.

After a fast we gasp at how salty, sour, spicy and/ or sweet we have grown to like our foods.

2. We lose weight.

It is not unusual to lose about a pound or two per day for the first few days, then one-half pound per day afterwards.

Sixty-two percent of our population — those who are overweight or obese — could improve their well-being by losing weight.

3. Our bodies are often healed.

Much healing takes place automatically during a fast. (More about this later). Our body gets into an excretion mode. Toxins of all kinds get released into the blood and are processed mainly by the kidneys, liver, skin, and lungs.

The immune system gets a boost in strength.

Your bowels function better after a fast.

Blood pressure, cholesterol, and fatty acid levels usually return to normal ranges during a fast of 14 days or longer. They will remain at normal readings if the person fasting modifies his eating and lifestyle habits. Otherwise, in four weeks or less all gain in health has been lost.

4. The mind becomes alert.

You are able to concentrate and remember things more acutely, especially in a fast of seven days or more.

5. Aging processes are slowed down.

You often look renewed and refreshed after a fast. Often times one sleeps more soundly.

6. Addictions give up.

If a fast of water continues long enough, the grip of unhealthy addictions will be broken. (This varies with individual genetics and habits.)

MY OWN EXPERIENCE WITH FASTING

Nearly 23 years ago I began to fast from after dinner on Friday until dinner on Saturday evenings. This taught me to humble myself before God.

As the Israelites said, "We afflicted our soul" (Isaiah 58:3 KJV).

Over time it gave my spirit strength to tell my body, mind, emotions, and will what I would or would not do, instead of allowing my body to control my spirit. That was one of the greatest possible benefits in those early days of fasting.

I started fasting on Saturdays because I was really hungry to know God better. I wanted to feel closer to God — to hear Him speak to me, if He wanted to. Also, I wanted to learn to pray more and more effectually.

Certainly these goals have been achieved to a satisfactory level. I believe I understood true repentance and true humility more after fasting for a few months. It caused me to become more God-conscious and less worldly minded, and I'm happy about that.

In addition, my health definitely improved. Some of the changes are only partially documented by medical records, but other things are clinically observable.

For example:

- My cholesterol level lowered from slightly above 200 to 154 in a relatively short period of time.
- My bad cholesterol count was down.
- My good cholesterol count was up, so I had less chance for heart disease.
- My tendency toward hypoglycemia leveled. I no longer have energy swings from high to low as I once did. I'm energetic all the time now.
- My tongue is never coated.
- My eyes are clear.
- My blood pressure is good.
- I don't have cravings or go on food binges anymore. Food isn't preeminent in my thinking all the time. I don't care about candy, doughnuts,

cakes, pies, ice cream, and many other poor nutrition foods. I truly do not!

- I've given up most of my caffeine, so my heart doesn't have irregular palpitations anymore.
- I'm hardly ever sick, as I've already said. I have a constant high level of physical and mental energy.
- I sleep well and feel rested when I awaken.

One medical doctor told me in 1996 after a complete physical (including a CAT scan), "Your blood is pure and your organs are clean. You are in better health than many young people who work in this hospital."

Later, I had a second complete examination at the Whitaker Wellness Clinic in Newport Beach, California. At the exit interview, I was told, "You have the bones of a 30-40 year-old woman." (I was 77 years old at the time.) "You and your secretary can make seven more trips around the world before you need to come back here."

Those excellent reports did not "just happen." My diet has gradually improved since 1980, when I was released from a life of total stress by retiring from my work. Also, I enjoyed moving to beautiful Arizona as opposed to the dark, dreary days of central Illinois. All of these events, I believe, contributed to my improved health.

MY 40-DAY FAST EXPERIENCE

From March 1 to April 9, 1998, I joined thousands — maybe millions — of Americans in a 40-day fast. Here is a list of my physical changes in symptoms.

1. The greatest healing that is visible involves my skin.

- The brown spots on the back of both hands are greatly diminished — not totally removed.
- "Old-age" spots on my forehead at my hairline are totally removed.
- Three small growths on my left eyelid are removed without a trace.
- The skin on my chest was rough and bumpy; it is now quite smooth.
- Scars on a finger and my right arm from an accident at five years of age are much less noticeable and much smoother in texture. An amazing difference!
- A "tag" of skin on the side of my nose is 90 percent healed.

2. My addiction to coffee is healed — even my first-thing-in-the-morning cup!

3. My ears underwent a healing as my nasal catarrh dried up almost completely (after years of suffering).

4. My liver, I believe, underwent a healing — judging from a pain in that area that lasted four days at around days 30-34 of the fast.

5. A fungus fingernail and toenail are back to normal.

6. I lost 15 pounds. My present weight is five pounds below what is desirable for my sex, height, age, and activity level.

7. A small fatty tumor is gone; a larger one is not as hard as before the fast, and it can be moved around easily.

8. On some days my eyesight is sharper — but not everyday. (I have macular degeneration).

Am I pleased with these physical fruits? Yes, more than pleased. I am grateful to God for giving me the strength to continue on the fast for the full 40 days.

Will this extend my life? I'm not even caring! I look better, feel better, think better, feel closer to God and more spiritually "tuned." Those benefits are rewards enough.

Take heart. You too can fast and receive health benefits if you decide to discipline yourself with fasting and prayer.

I bless you with the strength you need to enter into and practice this powerful spiritual tool.

DISEASES THAT YIELD TO FASTING

Hippocrates, the father of medicine, as well as Socrates and Plato, used fasting as a viable treatment modality to facilitate nature's self-healing processes for eliminating a large number of diseases. Modern doctors are just now accepting fasting in the same way. Here are a few examples.

People can fast away such conditions as allergies, asthma, bladder disease, bursitis, hay fever, high blood pressure, kidney disease, nervous exhaustion, obesity, poor circulation, rheumatism, schizophrenia, skin diseases, and stress.

Fasting is a successful treatment also for acne, anemia, appendicitis, arthritis, bronchitis, cirrhosis, colitis, constipation, diabetes, epilepsy, gallstones, glaucoma, goiter, gonorrhea, hemorrhoids, hepatitis, hypertension, insomnia, multiple-sclerosis, Parkinson's disease, peptic ulcers, sinusitis, tumors, and varicose veins.

The list goes on to include anxiety, cardiovascular diseases such as atherosclerosis and angina, Chrone's disease, chronic skin diseases such as psoriasis and eczema, depression, liver disease, lupus, migraine headaches, neurosis, and prostate problems.

If your disease is not listed here, do not give up hope. Almost all disease conditions can be benefited by fasting. Some doctors say cancer cannot be healed by fasting; other doctors disagree and testify to having success with cancer patients.

This list of conditions was compiled from several books, tapes, and a video that are listed in the bibliography.

CHAPTER THREE

Guidelines for Fasting

For a fast to be deemed successful, it must follow certain guidelines that include theoretical and practical knowledge for all three aspects of our nature — the spiritual, psychological, and physical. Why is that? Because all three of these parts comprising our whole being are, to some degree, "toxic."

We have fed ourselves junk and abused our bodies, minds, and spirits for years in many different ways. Fasting has been proven, I believe, as a viable procedure for bringing about a "dumping and cleansing" syndrome. Let me explain.

HOW TO PREPARE SPIRITUALLY

As was said in the introduction to this book, fasting and fitness are synonymous terms whether you are speaking spiritually, psychologically, or physically. Fasting, when done correctly, is a viable treatment modality for producing health as well as for preventing and/or reversing a whole host of illnesses — illnesses of the body, the soul, and the spirit.

Fasting will accomplish little of a lasting nature unless it is done as unto the Lord. So let's look at our decision to fast from God's point of view.

What would He have us accomplish on a fast? What spiritual goals would He have us set?

Here is a short list to stimulate our thinking:

1. God wants us to worship Him with all of our strength.

"O worship the Lord in the beauty of holiness: fear before him, all the earth" (Psalm 96:9 KJV).

Have American Christians learned to really worship the Lord? Since I have watched the Chinese underground believers worship, I have to say no.

Fasting is a good time to work on learning to worship God.

2. God wants us to daily model His character.

God is love, joy, peace, goodness, mercy, kindness, wisdom, holiness, patience, justice, grace, and faithfulness.

A fast is a good time for us to meditate on how closely our character is patterned after His character.

3. Ask God to show you how to become totally dependent on Him — for everything.

Any other position prevents the Spirit from operating. Total dependence is accomplished by abiding in the vine. (See John 15:4.)

Fasting aids in making us humble, and obtaining humility is a prerequisite for receiving God's best.

4. Learn to hate sin, love righteousness, fear God, and live a holy life.

Obedience to every word of God is the highest form of love. God is happy when we delight in walking in His ways instead of feeling obliged to do so out of fear or obligation.

5. God wants us to overcome strongholds in our lives.

Fasting is an incredible weapon for breaking down strongholds.

In Matthew 17:21, Jesus said, "However, this kind [demon] does not go out except by prayer and fasting" (NKJV).

A short list of strongholds might include: pride, self-centeredness, no fear of God, unforgiveness, apathy, lust, materialism, rebellion, anger, disobedience.

Ask God to show you your strongholds; we all have them. Spend some time before you fast learning how to pray effectively against these sins.

6. God's high calling for us is ministry — not achieving positions of authority or great power.

How are we doing in this area? God has gifted every person in unique ways to enable them to achieve His purposes in their lives. Ministry was in God's mind when we were just a thought yet to be created.

Multitudes of believers have not given enough thought concerning how God wants to use them. Neither have they found their true purpose and destiny in life! Ask God about this as you begin to fast.

7. Since love is the most powerful force in the world when it comes to influencing people for good, God desperately wants us to develop the art of loving.

His love never excludes, never limits, and never fails. That is the only kind of love He would like for us to exemplify. First Corinthians 13 is the biblical account given to us by the apostle Paul as a model for behaving lovingly.

FASTING IS GOOD NEWS

Fasting is one of the distinctive marks that should set Christians apart as servants of the Lord Jesus Christ.

The Jewish people understood fasting this way. Leviticus 16:29 says that on the day of atonement all Jewish people must "afflict their soul." From many centuries before Christ until this very day, the Jewish people have understood that to afflict your soul means to fast.

The great Bible teacher, Derek Prince, said, "It is a good thing to afflict your soul. If you are willing to do this for yourself, you will avoid many of the afflictions which God might otherwise have to bring upon you."[8]

In 1 Corinthians 11:31, Paul wrote that "if we would judge ourselves, we should not be judged [by the Lord]." Fasting is a way of judging yourself. It is afflicting your soul; it is humbling your soul; it is denying yourself.

In Matthew 16:24, Jesus says: "If any man will come after me, let him deny himself" (KJV).

The first step in following Christ is to "deny yourself." The egotistical self in you has to be denied. To deny means literally to say "no."

By fasting, you say "no" to your self-will and to your carnal appetites; you bring your soul into subjection to your spirit.

For the sincere, dedicated Christian, fasting is good news. It is a blessing — a privilege, not a burden or a hardship. Why is this true? Because fasting always brings its reward. It always opens up the will of God in your life; it always frees the Holy Spirit to do His work.

GETTING TO KNOW THE HOLY SPIRIT

As a way of ending this chapter, let me share with you a partial list of some of the many functions of the Holy Spirit. Perhaps it will challenge you to covet His friendship.

The Holy Spirit:

- Helps us. (See 1 Corinthians 2:10; John 14:26; Acts 8:26.)
- Convicts us. (See John 16:8; Romans 8:16.)
- Leads us. (See John 14:4; John 16:13; 1 John 2:27.)
- Empowers us. (See Acts 1:8; Romans 8:13-14; 1 Corinthians 12:8-11.)
- Liberates us. (See Romans 8:2; 2 Corinthians 3:17.)
- Seals us. (See Ephesians 1:13-15.)
- Prays for us. (See Romans 8:26-27.)
- Comforts us. (See John 15:26-27.)
- Quickens us. (See John 6:63.)
- Gives us life. (See John 16:13.)
- Tells us about the future. (See John 16:13.)
- Reveals hidden truth. (See Ephesians 3:3-6.)
- Strengthens us in the inner man. (See Ephesians 3:16.)
- Gives us hope. (See Romans 15:13.)

SOUL PREPARATION FOR FASTING

The mind, emotions, and will comprise the soul. What can be done before and during a fast in the soulish realm to properly prepare for it?

Let's begin with Psalm 35:13: "I humbled myself with fasting."

You probably recognize immediately that the soul is the willful, often rebellious, part of man. It is the proud, stubborn, self-sufficient part of us that needs humbling. The soul houses the mind, and our thoughts eventually control our destiny.

A small series of short sentences from an unknown author have had a great influence on my mind. Let me share it with you.

"Whatever they are in your life, it is these 'little things' that will make the difference:

- Your thoughts create your attitudes.
- Your attitudes create your actions.
- Your actions create your habits.
- Your habits create your character.
- Your character creates your destiny."

When applied to the question of fasting, those principles certainly get to the heart of the matter.

Your mind must say the first yes — "I want to learn to fast." If it speaks consistently and loudly enough, you will learn to fast, and you will get excellent results — the kind that build character and control the destiny of your physical, emotional, and spiritual health.

The main purpose of all fasting is to humble ourselves. This task originates in the soulish realm with the goal of seeking a closer relationship with the triune God.

Sacrificing food and drink is one way to acknowledge that we deeply desire something or someone else with great intensity. Our soul doesn't yield food and drink easily — regardless of the reason.

FASTING FOR THE RIGHT REASONS

What are some soulish problems that might serve as a springboard for serious prayer before, during, and after a fast? Let me ask a few questions that might prove helpful.

- Our tongue exposes what is in the inside of us. Do we bless people more than curse them with our spoken words?
- Are we perfectionists, demanding, critical, and judgmental by nature and in practice?
- Do we constantly stir up confusion and uproar in social settings?
- Is anger a trait that we are known to display on a regular basis?

- Do we scheme to use others to make us look good?
- Are we domineering — always trying to control and have the upper hand?
- Do we possess any of these traits: insecurity, jealousy, suspicious, intimidating, manipulating, fear of man more than God, untrustworthy, paranoid, rebellious, stubborn, arrogant, etc.?

All of these are "old man" traits that "new" men (and women) subjected to Jesus Christ through salvation by faith should diligently seek the help of the Holy Spirit to overcome. Remember, by faith and with God, all things are possible.

Jesus knew that some people would fast for the wrong reasons, so He addressed that subject in Matthew 6:1-18. When our hearts are not right, it is possible to fast from impure motives like these:

- To get attention.
- To fulfill a "religious ritual" or obligation.
- To improve your attractiveness.
- To prove your own will power and strength.
- To force God to answer a prayer request.

WHEN THE SOUL SAYS "YES"

Probably the foremost single reason why Christians today do not fast is because the church has not even mentioned the term from the pulpit for decades. The next significant reason is because "self-denial" as a concept does not fit into our present predominant philosophy of our society.

The American people today have espoused a very liberal view of life. We are encouraged from many sources to "do our own thing," "be our own person," "decide what we want and go get it — now."

This generation is enamored with the concepts of freedom of thought, freedom of speech, and freedom of behavior. Subjecting to a rigorous program of self-denial is unthinkable to many people today.

Indulging in one's self as first priority is, of course, totally incongruent with the spiritual goal of fasting. Fasting fits only with the ethic of "love God first, others second, and ourselves last." It is done for the purpose of subjugating our own fleshly desires, attitudes, and values to those of God. And God's ways are totally different! They are totally spiritual and designed to make us become like Him!

Before fasting, these thoughts must first get approval in the soulish realm. It is from there that the emotions and will say "yes" and the body lines up to get involved in the act. The spirit of man, of course, is now contented for he has known all along that it was God's will for men to honor Him with fasting.

ASK YOURSELF SOME QUESTIONS

Here are some suggestions to consider before you fast.

1. Determine the purpose of your fast.
Ask yourself these questions to determine your purpose and expose your true heart motives:

- Is it to get closer to God? (I pray so!)
- Is it to show humility and repentance?
- Do you want mainly to improve your general health?
- Could it be mainly for weight loss?
- Is there a specific illness you want to get rid of?
- To hear from God more clearly?
- To seek guidance for a special situation?
- For getting rid of an addiction?

All of these are legitimate reasons for fasting, but hopefully the major goal is for spiritual rather than physical or emotional enrichment.

2. Determine the length of your fast.
The length of your fast may well be determined by a number of factors:

- Your present state of health. The sicker you are, the shorter your first few fasts should last.

- Your work schedule. You need time to rest more while you are fasting.
- Think of a time during the week that would be best. When I worked as a university professor, Saturday was my day to fast. Find yours.
- Follow your divine guidance in this. If you are close to God, the Holy Spirit will answer your questions about when, how, and for how long.

In Scripture, those fasts where the time span is recorded were short in duration, usually one to three days. Other fasts of 7, 10, 21, and 40 days are also recorded. Even one day a week can make a tremendous spiritual difference in your life.

PREPARING YOUR BODY TO FAST

More and more health professionals are encouraging their patients to fast as a part of their treatment. At the same time, the procedures that these professionals recommend differ slightly, but in principle they are solidly together. Let me share the views of three persons.

Here is a compiled list of pre-fast recommendations:

- If you use coffee, tea, alcohol, cola drinks, or other stimulants, cut back or give them up a week or two before the fast.

- Move away from eating any animal protein (meat) at all a week or two before fasting.
- Begin to drastically lower your fat intake. Giving up all meat will help with this. Also decrease cheese, butter, margarine, oil, and foods prepared in these fats before you fast.
- Eat only fruits and vegetables for two or three days before fasting. Eat lots of green salads with chopped fresh vegetables.
- Eliminating all sugary products will greatly enhance the ease of fasting and its benefits.
- Pharmaceutical drugs need to be monitored during a fast; several weeks of one or two day fasts can often decrease the dosage needs for most drugs. A prolonged fast is then easier to accomplish.

WHAT HAPPENS WHEN YOU FAST?

1. Your metabolism changes.

The fact of the human body being "fearfully and wonderfully made" (Psalm 139:14) is again well illustrated when the energy metabolism in fasting humans is studied.

Vanderbilt University's School of Medicine did such a study in 1994, and the report is printed in the *American Journal of Clinical Nutrition,* (60:29-36). This study was characterized by being among the first to study all three major sources of fuel foods: carbohydrates, fats, and proteins simultaneously during a fast.

Their findings showed that the fasted state in humans demands a shift from using primarily starches and sugar foods (carbohydrates) as the main source of energy to the use of a fat-based fuel economy. This shift is by nature's design. Although it is very complex — even to the scientist — it is scientifically exquisite in every step of each process.

The burning of fat stores from many sources during fasting is a central component of the shift in fuel economy with fasting. We observe that everyone loses weight while fasting. The adipose tissue gives up free fatty acids, and they supply our energy for the majority of tissue needs.

One of the sources of fat made available for burning as fuel during an extended fast is from the inside of arteries and veins. The main component of atherosclerotic plaque is cholesterol — thus it is not surprising to learn that cholesterol levels are reduced by fasting.

The use of glucose, however, is still required for certain tissues, especially the brain. Glucose homeostasis (perfect balance) during a fast has been programmed into our cells for our protection during times of food deprivation. This study demonstrated that fact.

The volunteer subjects consumed only non-caffeine containing beverages of the no-energy type. Yet none of the subjects developed hypokalemia (low blood calcium), and none required oral potassium or other supplements.

There were significant changes in a number of energy metabolism processes:

- A six-fold increase in growth hormone production, the regulator of nocturnal (night time) metabolism of fats in humans.
- Glucagon, epinephrine, and norepinephrine concentrations doubled.
- Adipose tissue decomposition increased 2.5 fold.
- Fat oxidation (burning of fat) doubled, producing much greater production of ketones (mild acidosis condition). The kidneys filter the ketones, however, to prevent the blood from becoming too acidic.
- Plasma glucose concentrations decreased.
- Oxidation of glucose decreased.
- A decrease of plasma insulin concentrations took place.
- Free fatty acids tripled.
- Protein oxidation increased.

The biochemistry of all the alterations in normal fuel metabolism are impossible to describe to readers without a knowledge of chemistry. Suffice it to say that the increases and reductions in many involved substances during fasting metabolism illustrate a precise regulation that almost defies our imaginations.

How could all of these alterations take place without negatively affecting our daily functioning? That's a question to ask our Creator when we have the chance.

2. *The immune system improves.*

Another important physiological change during fasting would include an increase in the ability of white blood cells to destroy harmful bacteria. One explanation for this phenomena involves the total abstinence of sugar being ingested during the fast; the role of how sugar suppresses the body's ability to fight disease is widely known.

Still another way the immune system shows itself superior during a fast is in an increase in the antibody levels of IgA, IgM, and IgG — (three immunoglobulins that fight disease). Studies are available to explain the biochemical basis for the improvement of disease activity but seem inappropriate to include here.

3. *Toxins are dumped.*

All toxins are waste products for which the body cannot find a useful purpose. As a result, they put a tremendous burden on our organs. By diverting energy and nutrients from doing the tasks of repair, maintenance, and healing, toxins lower the body's ability to perform at peak levels for good health.

The "dumping toxins" syndrome is another physiological process that is well documented during times for fasting. Each cell has a "recipe" in its computer (nucleus) of how to dump waste into the connective tissues, blood and blood vessels, the lymphatic system (mesenchyme), etc. Apparently, God has pre-programmed our cells to eliminate toxins rapidly when we fast.

God meant for us to fast as a way of cleansing our cells. Fasting is God's way of keeping the body healthy so it can heal.

This description of the physiology of fasting is quite incomplete, yet I believe it is "enough said" for most readers. I am telling myself that it is better to say too little than too much. Hopefully I have made the right choice.

PHYSICAL SYMPTOMS WHILE FASTING

The symptoms are different with every fasting person. It seems the stronger you are physically and spiritually, the less trouble you will experience. If God asked you to fast, it's either "a piece of cake" all the way, or He wants to bring you through some

"Gethsemane moments" to test your sacrificial obedience.

Nevertheless, almost everyone experiences some changes that feel like symptoms. The commonly experienced ones would include:

- *Headaches.* These are usually the result of withdrawal from caffeine, alcohol, nicotine, food additives, and other drugs. Burning fats for energy can also produce headaches.
- *Vomiting.* This is the shortest route to the outside for toxins to be eliminated! It doesn't usually last too long. Should it persist, however, stop your fast.
- *Stomach aches.* This can be bile from the liver.
- *Coated tongue.* A white coverage shows release of toxins. This will go away if the fast continues long enough to fully cleanse you of metabolic waste.
- *Bad breath.* It smells like acetone — a sweet, fruity smell produced from incomplete oxidation of fats.
- *Dizziness.* This is usually caused by getting up from a sitting or lying position too quickly. It could be from low blood pressure but not usually in healthy individuals. It can also be caused by the liver cleansing.

- *Hunger.* This is a very normal reaction. Ask for God's help and sip lots of lemon water. It usually goes away in two to three days.

- *Cotton-mouth taste.* This is a good sign produced by detoxification.

- *A feeling of coldness.* Your heart is resting somewhat so not as much circulation is going on.

- *Tingling sensations.* These seem normal in some persons.

- *Tiredness.* This can be for many reasons; no caffeine or white sugar stimulation are two examples.

- *Fever.* May occur on an extended fast, but it is usually short lived.

- *Muscle soreness.* Often results from toxin release.

- *Moodiness.* Impatience, irritability, crankiness, self-pity, etc. are a possibility, especially at first.

- *Change in elimination.* No food means no elimination usually after the first day. It is not unusual, however, to experience diarrhea, especially the first few days. This results from toxins being dumped.

- *Loss of weight.* This is mostly water. Don't worry. Your weight will quickly return when you begin regular meals again.

CHOOSE YOUR FOODS CAREFULLY

My own study and experience with fasting spans a period of more than 22 years. In addition, I have accepted the advice of health professionals whose supervision of patients in their fasting clinics has allowed them to suggest specific guidelines. Special mention goes to the work of the late Dr. Julio Ruibal of Columbia, South America, and Dr. Joel Fuhrman of Belle Mead, New Jersey.

Here are my conclusions.

The way to end a fast is directly related to two major factors: (1) the kind of fast you undertook; (2) the length of your fast.

For those who engaged in a pure water fast, consulting with a certified health professional trained in fasting is highly recommended. For those who participated in a partial fast, the purer the food you ingested during your fast, the slower you should be in returning to normal eating.

Likewise, the longer the fast you were on, the more gradual should be your reintroduction of solid food. Let me explain.

Foods with the most to the least cleansing power can be ranked as follows:

- *Pure water* alone causes the greatest release of toxins from the cells and brings the greatest restoration of health.

- *Freshly squeezed fruit and vegetable juices* are great detoxifiers. All fruit juices (fresh, frozen, or bottled) should be diluted about 1/3 with water because of their high sugar content. Dr. Julio Ruibal highly recommended a vegetable juice drink drink of 1/3 carrot, 1/3 celery, and 1/3 dark green leaves (spinach, collards, kale, etc.). The electrolyte value of this drink is excellent and prevents problems often incurred in a long fast.
- *Vegetable broths* from a wide variety of cooked vegetables, including diluted bean juices, provide excellent cleansing and are a good source of water soluble vitamins and minerals. A combination of carrots, string beans, celery, zucchini, and parsley are excellent vegetables for "juice fasting" — or for breaking a fast.
- *Raw fruits and/or raw vegetables* are good cleansers. Apples, oranges, watermelon, pears, grapes, etc., plus zucchini, asparagus, string beans, and carrots are good foods to use.
- *Cooked fruits and vegetables* rank only fourth.
- *Grains, beans, and legumes* — any whole grain. The higher fiber in these cleanse the colon.
- *Non-cleansing foods* such as meats, eggs, cheese, sugars, cola beverages, etc. are the last foods to add when coming off a fast. Always eat less and less of these items in your new "regular diet."

Being a total vegetarian has many health benefits. (See Genesis 1:29.)

HOW TO BREAK A SHORT FAST

For fasts of one to three days, the matter of breaking the fast is not as crucial as when the length of the fast has been seven days and beyond. You may return immediately to your regular pattern of eating by using wisdom and common sense about the amount of food ingested at one meal. Eat with temperance and listen to your body's signal for when enough is enough.

Avoid huge meals, fatty foods, lots of meat, and sugary foods and beverages. This should be your new lifestyle anyway. Fresh fruits and lots of fresh vegetables are always healthful, especially at the end of a fast. They keep you from another toxic build-up.

Here is a suggested pattern for returning to normal meals.

- *For Breakfast:* Give yourself a medium-sized serving of 2-3 fresh fruits (1/2 banana, 1/2 apple, 1/2 grapefruit, for example). That starts the enzymes and simple digestive juices.

    Freshly squeezed juices would also be excellent. A serving of BarleyGreen adds lots of good nutrition (16 vitamins, 23 minerals, 18 amino acids, about 300 enzymes, chlorophyll which is a healer, and an alkaline pH — another healer). All of this for 10 calories per teaspoon.

- *For Lunch:* A baked sweet potato as the main dish would be excellent. A few bites of other fresh vegetables (raw or slightly steamed) would be good. Keep control of the size of the servings. Purified water with lemon to drink — no ice!

- *For Dinner:* A serving of brown rice with nice-sized servings of two or three additional vegetables. Whole wheat bread is all right now. More lemon water to drink.

HOW TO BREAK AN EXTENDED FAST

The way to break a fast of seven days or more and return to normal eating is very important. During fasting, you have caused physiological rest of all organs, glands, tissues, and systems (endocrine, hormonal, enzymatic, digestive, nervous, cardiovascular, lymphatic, muscular, respiratory, circulatory, etc.). Many processes — like digestion, assimilation, and elimination — have been "sleeping."

For digestion to begin, the enzymatic system must produce between 2,000-3,000 enzymes. It must produce digestive juices, which takes time, energy, and nutrients galore. Give your body time to get up to speed — about three days. Otherwise you will produce internal stress that can make you ill, very ill, in fact.

Digestion is a very complex process. It takes time and energy to get meat, vegetables, fruits, grains, and dairy products — not to mention all the junk food — into our bloodstream where the vitamins, minerals, sugars, starches, amino acids (proteins), and fatty acids can be used. It requires attention also to proper techniques for eating food.

Your intestines are also "sleepy." Don't jerk them out of their slumber and stress them with lots of waste to handle. They don't function "half asleep" any better than you do!

These are my recommendations based on the works of several health professionals, including M.D.s.

Looking at the list of foods with the most to the least cleansing power, it follows logically that if you were on a pure water only fast, you should be the longest at getting back to normal eating — three or four days is recommended.

There are a few other "do's and don'ts" that should be followed:

- Eat small amounts of food for several days.
- Eat small bites at a time.
- Chew your food until it is almost a cream before swallowing it.
- Limit your meals to no more than three items. Digestive enzymes and juices must be manufactured for each different food. Keep meals simple.

- Do not rinse each bite or two down with a beverage; this dilutes the juices that are working on digestion.
- Do not drink iced beverages. The body has to heat them before they can function, and that takes energy — energy needed for digestion.
- After three days (for healthy persons) or four days (for unhealthy persons), you may return to normal eating. Your body will help you know the right time — if you listen carefully.

HOW TO BREAK AN EXTENDED WATER FAST

After a water fast, follow these rules:

- *Day 1:* Drink freshly squeezed fruit and/or vegetable juices (with carrot base) and take Barley-Green every two hours, if you like.
- *Day 2:* Eat small servings of fresh fruits every 2-3 hours, again, with BarleyGreen. Watermelon and oranges are excellent.
- *Day 3:* More of the same with homemade vegetable broth. One quart per day is a good amount.
- *Day 4:* Have any of the above plus some steamed vegetables.

Meals on day 3 or 4 might look something like this:

- *For Breakfast:* An orange or a piece of water-melon are ideal. You may have these foods every two hours, if you feel the need.[9] Barley-Green (1-2 tsp.) in juice or freshly squeezed apple, orange, or grapefruit juice. Drink lots of lemon water all day, not with ice.

- *For Lunch:* Have a small baked sweet potato as your main course with a few bites of some light-ly steamed or raw fresh vegetables. Eat only small amounts. Drink lemon water.

- *For Dinner:* Have a vegetable plate of three medium-sized servings of vegetables. To drink Barley-Green 30 minutes before each meal or between meals is good.

Again, omit iced beverages from your meals since the body needs to heat them before they can function, and this takes energy away from digestion.

When the body gets thoroughly chilled, the functions of the digestive system (and others also) are slowed down. The pulse rate and circulation are slower, respiration is depressed, toxic waste stays in the tissues longer, and the whole organism functions poorly. This is a definite stress situation. Be sure to put on more clothes, and do what you need to do to get and keep a normal temperature.

IF YOU OVEREAT TOO QUICKLY

A friend recently fasted for 25 days on a juice fast. He broke his fast by having a meal consisting only of four steamed vegetables: carrots, small potatoes, broccoli, and spinach — no butter added, no bread, etc.

He became so ill that he was forced to leave work and go to bed for the rest of the day. He was nauseated (but did not vomit), was very dizzy, had a headache, felt totally without strength and vitality. His intestines cramped for several hours, and all he wanted to do was sleep. My friend overtaxed his "sleepy digestive system," and it was quick to complain!

When you overeat too soon after a fast, stomach cramps, vomiting, and a general feeling of malaise are common symptoms.

Another strong suggestion. Go easy on spicy foods like black pepper, pickles, mustard, and such. The mucosal defense barrier in the stomach has been weakened; it takes time for it to be built back to normal.

Here is my blessing to all fasters who need to get back to normal eating:

In the Name of Jesus, I bless you with the power to always eat for good health the rest of your life. As you follow God's plan for eating and fasting, may the Lord remove from you all sickness and make your body immune to modern deadly diseases. Amen.

COMPLICATIONS FROM FASTING

This list of possible complications from fasting has been taken from several sources — mostly from my own class lecture notes. (See the bibliography since I am unable to give credit for these items.)

- *Hypoglycemia:* Deficiency of sugar in the blood.
- *Impaired glucose intolerance:* Glucose is a sugar and also an intermediate in metabolism of carbohydrates that are formed during digestion.
- *Ketosis:* The accumulation in the body of the ketone bodies. (Ketone bodies are a group of compounds produced during the oxidation of fatty acids.)
- *Lactic acidosis:* Lactic pertains to milk. Acidosis is a disturbance in the acid-base balance of the body in which there is an accumulation of acids.
- *Hyperuricemia:* An abnormal amount of uric acid in the blood.
- *Loss of nitrogen:* Nitrogen is one of the important elements in all proteins, essential for tissue building.

- *Lean tissue:* Tissue is a group or collection of similar cells that act together in the performance of a particular function.
- *Hypoalanimeia and hair loss:* Results from not enough alanine — an amino acid.
- *Loss of potassium, sodium, calcium, magnesium, and phosphate.*
- *Reduced kidney function:* The kidney excretes urine that contains end products of metabolism and helps regulate the water, electrolyte, and acid base content of the blood.
- *Edema:* A condition in which the body tissues contain an excessive amount of tissue fluid.
- *Anuria:* Complete urinary suppression or kidney failure.
- *Hypotension:* Decrease of blood pressure below normal.
- *Anemia:* A reduction in number of red blood cells or in hemoglobin.
- *Alterations in liver function:* Liver stores and metabolized carbohydrates, fats, and proteins and helps detoxify many poisonous substances that may be ingested.
- *Decreased serum iron binding capacity:* Serum pertains to fluid.
- *Gastrointestinal tract changes:* Pertains to stomach and intestines.
- *Nausea and vomiting.*

- *Alteration in thyroxine metabolism and impaired serum triglyceride metabolism:* Thyroxine relates to thyroid hormone; triglyceride relates to most animal and vegetable fats.

From this list of potential health problems, it is easy to deduct that fasting sometimes requires close supervision of a trained health professional.

A list of experienced doctors in the field of fasting and also a list of fasting clinics is found in Appendix A. We acknowledge that neither list is exhaustive.

WHAT ABOUT TAKING MEDICATION?

The average person my age (78), I am told, is on five or six drugs — for heart, joints, diabetes, high blood pressure, and a whole list of other diseases. Should they go on a fast and continue their medications?

The facts are that most people can be liberated from taking their medications when they have proper food, get some exercise, enough sleep, and spend time meditating on inspired writings, i.e., the Scriptures, for stress management. It is not a simple matter, however, and it requires the help of a qualified health professional.

My experience in helping others with this situation is to recommend a primarily fresh fruit and vegetable diet with modest servings of whole grains, nuts, and seeds for a month or even more before beginning a fast.

Two to four teaspoons of BarleyGreen each day goes a long way in starting the "detox/repair/heal" processes. Many times the dosage of medications can then be decreased without a problem.

Even with these preparations, it is good to be checked by your doctor before actually beginning a fast. While you are fasting, your body may let you know that it needs less medication.

If you seek the help of a fasting clinic physician, of course, the matter soon becomes a moot point; their experience often leads you safely to a drug-free situation.

WHAT ABOUT TAKING SUPPLEMENTS?

While I believe in supplementation to offset the inferior American diet, I do not recommend continuing your regimen while you are fasting. Why is that? Because vitamins, minerals, digestive enzymes, amino acids, and other nutrition elixirs all require food for them to be absorbed and to do their work. If there is no food in the stomach, the addition of these nutrients can only cause stress and discomfort.

Have you ever taken your vitamins on an empty stomach before going to work or school without breakfast? And did you feel a little nauseated on the way?

My advice: Do not take your vitamins and mineral supplements or other nutrition preparations while fasting. But again, ask your doctor.

FASTING AND YOUR COLON

Dr. Dennis Burkitt of South Africa gave a lecture years ago concerning the problem of impacted and encrusted fecal matter in the colons of Americans — a problem nonexistent in Africans. Why? Americans do not eat enough fiber in their diet.

What happens to the fiber in our grains? During a visit to a cereal manufacturing plant, I learned how all layers of bran are removed from the grains being brought to the factory from surrounding farms. Six layers of bran — the brooms God designed so perfectly to sweep fecal matter through the intestinal tract while providing niacin, pyridoxine, pantothenic acid, riboflavin, thiamine, and protein — are all stolen from the American people. Where does the valuable bran go? Into farm animal formulas!

What has been the result? An epidemic of parasites, of many varieties, in the colon — even among our children. Plaque-coated intestines provide the perfect milieu for worms, resulting in a whole host of parasitic diseases — often missed by the medical profession in diagnosis.

In addition, the lack of fiber in the American diet has increased those troubled by diverticulosis, colon spasms, appendicitis, hemorrhoids, constipation, and colon cancer.

What happens to the colon during a fast? After the first or second day, nothing. Elimination stops. That is normal and should not cause concern. Normal bowel movements usually return one to two days after the eating of regular meals is resumed.

Should one take enemas or colonics during the fast? Some authors say yes; others, no. Coffee enemas are believed to be helpful by some; colonics are favored by others.

I like what Dr. Paul C. Bragg recommended. Before a fast, daily take 1-3 teaspoonfuls of equal parts of oat-bran and psyllium husk powder added to your drinks, soups, hot cereals, or other foods for a few days. "Thousands have reported good results by adding this inexpensive mixture to their diet."[10]

IS FASTING SAFE FOR EVERYONE?

No, fasting, unfortunately, is not for everyone. The following people should not fast:

- Extremely thin people in very poor health.
- Extremely weak people.
- People with known kidney or liver damage.

- People with cancer of the liver, kidneys, or pancreas.
- People with advanced stages of heart disease, where breathing is very labored.
- People recuperating from surgery or accidents.
- Pregnant or lactating women should not go on an extended fast.
- Type 1 diabetic patients cannot fast.

This list is not exhaustive. Ask your doctor if you have doubts about whether or not you should fast.

MAKE FASTING A WAY OF LIFE

Hopefully you have learned that fasting is a natural physiological process that nature built into the animal kingdom — at least in rhinoceroses, elephants, dogs, cats, etc. When an animal feels "under the weather," the appetite scoots! When wellness returns, so does the desire for food.

Fasting is also natural for human beings as a way of periodically cleansing the body of toxins and disease. Most health professionals who deal with fasting, however, advise only one 40-day fast per year.

You have also learned that fasting is a biblical concept that began in Genesis and persists until today — not only in Christianity but other world religions as well.

As you read the benefits of fasting to the spirit, the soul, and the body, which improvement would you like never to experience again? If your answer is none of them, then I have another question. Why not make fasting a regular part of your lifestyle — one day a week, one meal a day, or any other pattern that fits your lifestyle? Because, yes:

- Your health will return to you speedily.
- Your righteousness will go before you.
- You will cry and God will answer you.
- The Lord will guide you continually.
- You will be like a well-watered garden.

And much, much more. (See Isaiah 58:8-12.)

CHAPTER FOUR

God's Plan for Health

To help readers of this book understand my confidence in making dietary recommendations, let me share my personal story.

SICK MICE CONVINCED ME!

Years ago, as a student working in Ohio State University's Nutrition Research laboratory, I saw firsthand the direct response of dietary deficiencies and dietary alterations on experimental animals, especially white mice.

Facts established by well-controlled research on laboratory animals show many relationships between poor nutrition and health.

Examples are:

- Stunted growth
- Dry, scaly skin
- Bad blood
- Weeping eyes
- Rotten teeth
- No appetite
- No vigor
- Nervous temperaments
- Infections galore
- Porous bones

This "seeing is believing" experience made me want to know more about how to feed myself and my family. I knew good nutrition would result in better health and vitality, to say nothing of longevity with relative freedom from sickness and disease. After seeing the direct effects of prolonged under-nutrition on small animals and humans, I didn't want those conditions to afflict us.

OVEREATING YET UNDERNOURISHED

From that day until this, my interest in nutrition has grown from a local and national interest to an international concern. My travels have shown me the facts. Millions of people on this planet have emaciated bodies and stunted minds because of an insufficient or inadequate food intake.

Contrarily, in my own country the effects of *over-nutrition* are observable everywhere. According to a U.S. Public Health Survey, 62 percent of our population is now overweight. It is my belief that neither of these conditions, hunger or overweight, is good. Neither should continue.

Malnourished means being sick to one degree or another. Likewise, being overweight or obese creates chronic health problems.

- *Overweight* is defined as 10 to 19 percent above your ideal weight.
- *Obese* means being 20 percent or more above ideal weight.

To avoid the inevitable ill health that follows poor diets over a long period of time, many of us need a nutrition "conversion experience." We need to change our eating habits. We need to restrain our appetites and our taste buds. *That* will not be easy.

Our appetites need to be "born-again" — literally transformed and made new. It is wonderful for us to bring glory to God even through our eating and drinking.

It is obvious that making wise food choices and providing nutritious meals for yourself and your family become more complex and more expensive. Truly, the choices are difficult.

It's not only *how much* Americans eat, it's also *what* many people eat. Highly refined and "super-sweet" foods have flooded our supermarkets, and Americans are eating more and more of them.

As a nation we have also increased our intake of fats, especially saturated fats. Our relative state of affluence has permitted and encouraged an increase in the consumption of meats, particularly red meats. At the same time, we have chosen to decrease our consumption of fruits, vegetables, and whole-grain cereals. We have substituted many less-nutritious beverages, including soft drinks and alcoholic beverages, in place of drinking water.

These changes in our diets have been detrimental to health. For example, the over-consumption of meat, fast food, sugar, cholesterol, salt, and alcohol has been linked with a higher incidence in six of the ten leading causes of death in the United States: heart disease, cancer, cerebro-vascular disease, diabetes, arteriosclerosis, and hypertension.

Believe me on the basis of my 62 years of study and experience in this field. If we buy foods only from the *farm*acy, we will almost never need the services of the *pharmacy!*

THE GENESIS 1:29 CURE

Our diets should be changed by forsaking foods that have been produced by scientists (mankind) and return to the foods created for us by God Himself. What man or committee of men could possibly know as much about agriculture and horticulture as our Creator?

On the third day of creation, God created man's food supply and announced that it was good.

"And God said, Let the earth bring forth grass, the herb yielding seed, and the fruit tree yielding fruit after his kind, whose seed is in itself, upon the earth; and it was so" (Genesis 1:11 KJV).

Genesis 1:29 gave very clear directions to Adam and Eve as to how to eat: "And look! I have given you the seed-bearing plants throughout the earth, and all the fruit trees for your food" (TLB).

This statement was made by God to Adam and Eve. The original diet God planned for man is what we would call "a vegetarian diet."

Within the past 10 or 20 years, almost all researchers in nutrition have come to agree on these with God's plan:

- Americans need more fruits, more vegetables, more beans, lentils, legumes, and more *whole* (as opposed to processed/boxed) grains (cereals).
- Americans need less meat, milk, cheese, and eggs.
- Americans need much, much less sugar and fat.

Live food makes live people; dead food makes dead people. Re-read that statement and meditate on it for a minute or two. What is live food? Any food from the *farm*acy — which is any food created by God for human consumption.

What is dead food? Any food that man has de-natured by removing parts for the purpose of changing the original form of it. For example, fresh ears of corn are nothing like cornflakes. Wheat berries from the field do not resemble, nutritionally, white flour at all. White flour is a dead food; whole wheat is a plant "beefsteak"! And so it goes with thousands of possible illustrations.

DO'S AND DON'TS OF BIBLICAL NUTRITION

Let's read Genesis 1:29 from *The Living Bible:* "And he said, "Let the earth burst forth with every sort of grass and seed-bearing plant, and fruit trees with seeds inside the fruit, so that these seeds will produce the kinds of plants and fruits they came from.""

What foods fall into the categories God created for us to eat?

- *All beans/legumes/lentils/seeds and nuts.* (These should be your main sources of protein).
- *All whole grains:* barley, rice, wheat, oats, millet, corn, spelt, rye, quinoa, amaranth — any natural grain.

- *All fresh vegetables and fruits.* (Eat as many of them raw as you can tolerate. Frozen or canned vegetables and fruits are better than none!)
- *Distilled or reverse osmosis water only.* (6-8 glasses daily; this is very important.) Use fresh lemon in it to move your pH toward alkalinity.
- *Eat a wide variety of vegetables and fruits and whole grains.* The wider the variety, the better. This is the key to disease prevention and/or cure.

It takes only about eight months to one year to turn sick cells into healthy cells. For that to happen, you need to limit drastically or to omit totally the following foods:

- *All meat.* Omit *all* flesh, including fish and fowl, and especially pork. Pork is about 50 percent toxin, the "dirtiest" meat one can consume!
- *All whole milk products* — unless you can buy certified, unpasteurized milk. (See Proverbs 27:27.) Soy milk is good.
- *Eggs* — unless you can buy fertile farm eggs, and then only three to five per week.
- *"Man-made" products of all kinds.* "Designer foods" like artificial whipped cream are dead foods. Dead foods make dead people.
- *Most canned goods.* Naturally a few won't kill you.

- *All white sugar and baked goods using white flour.* Use whole wheat flour and honey, maple syrup, molasses, fruit juice concentrates, dates and raisins, etc. to sweeten.
- *All fruit juices except freshly squeezed ones.* Most have too much sugar for sick cells unless you dilute them about one-third to one-half with water.
- *Eat no margarine.* This "plastic-like" substance plugs arteries. Butter is okay in small amounts.
- *Water from your tap.* Chlorine and heavy metals produce free-radicals that produce carcinogens.
- *High-fat foods.* These include all fried foods, sandwich meats (like bologna, etc.), mayonnaise, snack foods, nuts in large amounts, doughnuts, potato and other chips, etc.
- *No oils* — other than cold-pressed virgin olive oil or safflower oil in cooking.
- *Coffee.* Drink no more than 1-2 cups per day; none if you have cancer. Use hot water with a slice of lemon instead. This will help cleanse the liver, kidneys, and bladder.

Of course, rest, exercise, and a positive mental attitude are also very important components of a healthy lifestyle.

HOW SCIENCE AND SCRIPTURE AGREE

It has taken scientists, as a group, about 6,000 years to agree with Scripture on the subject of foods and nutrition. Here is a quick summary of ways known to me about this subject.

Science says: Eat a wide variety of foods.

Scripture says: "Then God said, 'Let the earth bring forth grass, the herb that yields seed, and the fruit tree that yields fruit according to its kind, whose seed is in itself, on the earth'; and it was so" (Genesis 1:11 NKJV).

God gave this first principle of nutrition concerning His plan for man's food supply the third day of creation; and God saw that it was good.

The sixth day of creation, God made Adam and Eve and spoke to them about their diet. "And God said, 'See, I have given you *every* herb that yields seed which is on the face of all the earth, and *every* tree whose fruit yields seed; to you it shall be for food'" (Genesis 1:29 NKJV; italics mine).

All grains, beans, lentils, nuts, seeds, fruits, and vegetables were created and given to man for his sustenance and enjoyment. Indeed God meant for us to eat a wide variety of foods. Perhaps it is scientific to say that one of the main reasons our population today is so epidemically ill is because we are failing to regularly eat a wide variety of foods.

Science says: Maintain ideal weight.

Scripture says: Jesus said, "'And take heed to yourselves, lest at any time your hearts be overcharged with surfeiting [overeating], and drunkenness [over drinking], and cares of this life, and so that day come upon you unaware'" (Luke 21:34 KJV).

"When you sit down to eat with a ruler, consider carefully what is before you; And put a knife to your throat if you are a man given to appetite. Do not desire his delicacies, for they are deceptive food" (Proverbs 23:1-3 NKJV). (See also Psalm 141:3-4.)

"'But Jeshurun grew fat and kicked; You grew fat, you grew thick, you are covered with fat; Then he forsook God who made him, and scornfully esteemed the Rock of his salvation'" (Deuteronomy 32:15 NKJV).

Yes, eating is a spiritual matter!

"'When you have eaten and are full — then beware, lest you forget the Lord who brought you out of the land of Egypt, from the house of bondage'" (Deuteronomy 6:11-13 NKJV). "'When you are full, don't forget to be reverent to him and to serve him" (TLB).

These verses warn against overeating, which yields fatness of body and leanness of soul. Science and the Bible agree again!

Science says: Avoid too much fat, saturated fat, and cholesterol.

Scripture says: "'This shall be a perpetual statute throughout your generations in all your dwellings:

you shall eat neither fat nor blood'" (Leviticus 3:17 NKJV).

"'Speak to the children of Israel, saying: You shall not eat any fat, of ox or sheep or goat'" (Leviticus 7:23 NKJV).

"'The person who eats it shall be cut off from his people'" (Leviticus 7:25 NKJV).

How are people "cut off" today? By heart attacks, cancer, obesity, and a whole host of modern-day diseases so prevalent in America.

"He who loves wine and oil will not be rich" (Proverbs 21:17 NKJV). Why? Because of his shortened life span!

"'You shall not boil a young goat in its mother's milk'" (Deuteronomy 14:21 NKJV). Why? It produces a double saturated fat situation.

Many Scriptures mention using olive oil, which is a mono-saturated oil of highest quality. See Leviticus 2:4-7, 14:10, and 14:24 as examples.

Scientists have endorsed the use of olive oil in recent years as the most healthful fat.

Butter is also a biblically approved fat to eat. "And it shall come to pass, for the abundance of milk that they shall give he shall eat butter: for butter and honey shall every one eat that is left in the land" (Isaiah 7:22 KJV).

Meats can be as much as 40-60 percent fat, so Proverbs 23:30 is excellent advice: "Be not among winebibbers; among riotous eaters of flesh" (KJV). Riotous means "without constraint."

Scientists say 12 ounces of meat per week more than adequately meets one's need for protein. That would be less than 40 pounds per year; our present intake is at 275 pounds per year.

Our high cholesterol problem among Americans could be eliminated almost overnight just by following the Genesis 1:29 diet or by being obedient to any or all of the above verses.

Science says: Eat food with adequate starch and fiber.

Scripture says: The Genesis 1:29 diet (see above) — all grains, beans, lentils, nuts, seeds, fruits and vegetables — when eaten in a "wide variety" pattern is an excellent balance of all major and minor nutrients, including adequate fiber.

Scientists have concluded that the ideal combination of foods in a day's meals yields:

- 10-15 percent of calories in protein;
- 20-25 percent of calories in fat;
- 60-70 percent of calories in carbohydrates.

When eating whole, fresh, organically grown, unprocessed foods, you not only have the ideal amount of major nutrients but also an adequate fiber content for proper elimination of digestive waste. God's plan for man's health is like every other thing He created — exquisite in design and perfect in function.

In our diet today, we must consciously seek those unprocessed grains and daily eat our vegetables and fruits to assure we have adequate starch and fiber.

Science says: Avoid too many sweets.

Scripture says: "My son, eat honey because it is good, and the honeycomb which is sweet to your taste" (Proverbs 24:13 NKJV).

Proverbs 25:16 also has an important message. "Have you found honey? Eat only as much as you need, lest you be filled with it and vomit" (NKJV). (See also Proverbs 25:27.)

The problem of totally denatured sugar cane and sugar beets in the form of white sugar is not biblically addressed since it is a relatively new product (early 1800s). God made cane and beets to contain over 50 nutrients in each; white sugar (man's product) has zero nutrients. Americans at the turn of this century were consuming less than 10 pounds of sugar annually; we now consume around 130 pounds.

God must be saying to us, *"Too much! Too much!"*

Psalm 141:4 speaks of restricting the eating of too many "dainties." This probably includes high-sugar desserts and even the overeating of natural sweets like dates, raisins, and dried fruits as well as rich sauces and much wine.

Proverbs 23:3 defines "dainties" as deceitful meat.

The theologian, Adam Clarke, as long ago as the early 1800s, noted, "They [dainties] please but do not profit. They are pleasant to the sight, the smell and taste; but they are injurious to health."[11]

"Curds and honey He shall eat, that He may know to refuse evil and choose the good" (Isaiah 7:15 NKJV). Curds here refer to butter.

"Jonathan stretched out the end of the rod . . . dipped it in a honeycomb, and put his hand to his mouth; and his countenance brightened" (1 Samuel 14:27 NKJV).

Science says: Cut down on salt and foods high in salt.

Scripture says: "Can flavorless food be eaten without salt?" (Job 6:6 NKJV).

"'Every offering must be seasoned with salt, because the salt is a reminder of God's covenant'" (Leviticus 2:13 TLB).

According to 2 Kings 2:20-22, impure water was purified by the addition of salt and, in addition, the women ceased to have miscarriages and deaths decreased.

Luke 14:34 and Mark 9:50 say, "Salt is good."

The Bible does not contain a verse concerning the effects of too much salt. Scientific literature, however, supports the ill effects, including high blood pressure, dropsy, strokes, and nephritis. Present day intake of salt is considered to be excessive. Americans eat too many salted snack foods, pickles, salted meats, and nuts.

Science says: If you drink alcohol, do so in moderation.

Scripture says: "Wine is a mocker, intoxicating drink arouses brawling, and whoever is lead astray by it is not wise" (Proverbs 20:1 NKJV).

"Destruction is certain for that city — the pride of a people brought low by wine" (Isaiah 28:1 NLT).

"Woe to men mighty in drinking wine, woe to men valiant for mixing intoxicating drink" (Isaiah 5:22 NKJV).

"Do not mix with winebibbers, or with gluttonous eaters of meat; for the drunkard and the glutton will come to poverty" (Proverbs 23:20-21 NKJV).

"Do not look on the wine when it is red.... At the last it bites like a serpent, and stings like a viper" (Proverbs 23:30-32 NKJV).

Pediatricians until 1986 had a lenient policy regarding pregnant women and wine consumption. Their advice was: If you are accustomed to a glass of wine with dinner, go ahead and have it during pregnancy.

Then because of low birth-rate babies, newborns with birth defects, "poor start" in life babies (colicky children), the policy was changed to no wine for pregnant women.

An angel of the Lord came to Manoah (the father of Samson) and gave him this command concerning his expectant wife: "She may not eat anything that comes from the vine, nor may she drink wine or similar drink, nor eat anything unclean [non-Kosher]. All that I commanded her, let her observe" (Judges 13:14 NKJV).

It took scientists nearly 2,000 years to confirm the scriptural reference given plainly in Judges. Now we can say that science and the Bible agree on the advisability of avoiding wine and alcoholic beverages during pregnancy.

Yes, we have a health crisis in our country. It is absolutely related to our dietary habits. Our present sick population will never, never return to health until we forsake our present eating habits and return to God's *farm*acy.

I bless you with the strength you need to change your way of eating.

NATURE'S PILLS AND CAPSULES

Did you ever hear the words, "More than anything I want you to prosper and be in health, even as your mind, emotions and will [soul] prospers"? Let me help you get a new understanding of how serious God was when He inspired the apostle John to write very similar words to those in 3 John, verse 2. Let me explain.

Vitamins, minerals, carbohydrates, protein, and fats have been serious subjects of study, especially since the turn of the 20th century. Until 1988, however, scant research was done on the subject of phytochemicals (plant chemicals). Today the subject of phytochemicals has opened an exciting frontier that will bring breakthroughs in health for years to come.

Scientists have recently (since 1988) discovered over 20,000 new phytochemicals in fresh foods.

- *All* are medicines.
- *All* prevent or reverse disease.
- *None* may ever be sold in bottles or pills.

Phytochemicals, which can heal our sick cells, must be ingested in our daily meals.

Would you like to add years to your life and life to your years? You can. Get serious about ingesting nature's pills and capsules every time you eat. Your body — and your health — will be surely, but slowly, transformed.

ABOUT PHYTOCHEMICALS

What are phytochemicals and how do they act? Phytochemicals are:

- The plant's immune system.
- Perfect foods for us.
- God's choice of food for Adam and Eve. (See Genesis 1:29.)

Phytochemicals protect plants:

- From disease.
- Against injuries, insects, poisons, and pollutants in the air and soil.
- Against droughts and excessive heat, as well as ultraviolet rays.

Phytochemicals:

- Deter disease in animals and humans.
- Boost our immune system.
- Perform like doctors, nurses, surgeons, and "miracle healers" on the inside of us.

Plant chemicals work in various ways — probably many of which are yet to be discovered and understood. Here is a start at understanding what they have been found to do:

- Lower cholesterol when it's high.
- Lower blood pressure.
- Stimulate regular heartbeats.
- Detoxify the blood.

- Rebuild broken-down kidneys and livers.
- Heal ulcers and skin sores.
- Relieve allergies.
- Relieve any "itis" — arthritis, tonsillitis, bursitis, tendinitis, appendicitis.
- Improve memory.
- Reduce deafness and ringing in the ears.
- Alleviate depression and sexual impotency.
- Help detect and deter tumors, cancers, warts, and polyps.
- They battle the flu, pneumonia, all childhood diseases, and every conceivable disease.

NATURE'S DRUGS AND CHEMOTHERAPY

It should be obvious to Americans that the drugs and chemotherapies offered by our pharmaceutical companies are not healing very many people. In fact, two international studies have clearly shown that patients with cancer who take no drugs or chemotherapy live about as long — with fewer side-effects and as good or better quality of life — as those who submit to today's treatment modalities.

Be certain about one thing: *There is a remedy for cancer* — many remedies, in fact. All of them emanate from nature — and not from chemical factories and man-made drugs, in my opinion.

What can nature's remedies do?

- They can take tumors and defuse them. Some have antioxidant properties that keep the unstable molecules known as free radicals from wreaking cellular damage.
- Some seem to prevent the formation of carcinogens.
- Some block carcinogens from reaching their targets (cells). They can turn off the process of cancer.
- Some boost the production of enzymes that have a detoxifying effect on them. But these anticancer effects are just the tip of the iceberg.
- Other compounds appear to lower blood cholesterol and boost immune function.
- Carotenoids may enhance immune function and help prevent, or possibly reverse, osteoporosis as well.
- Some inhibit estrogen-promoted cancers such as in breast cancer by blocking them from reaching their targets.
- Some interfere with the production of estrogen.
- Some have the ability to enhance the liver's ability to inactivate estrogens.
- Some reduce blood cholesterol and many more things.

THE QUAD-COLOR DIET

Since my days at Ohio State University (1937-1940), I have known that the color of fruits and vegetables (as well as color in the whole universe) was very significant in regard to health. Now authors are writing about the "Tri-Color Chart"; the colors included there are green, orange/yellow, and red.

My color chart would need to be called "The Quad-Color Diet" because the fourth major color of fruits and vegetables is white. Here are a few words about each major color.

Let's begin with green.

1. Green Vegetables: Real Healers

Chlorophyll exhibits an incredible engineering feat on the part of nature. The chlorophyll in the grass is the blood of the plant. It is made from soil, air, water, and the sun.

Chlorophyll is the plant's source of life; without it, no plant survives. You can witness for yourself that without sunlight, air, and water, the leaves of all plants turn yellow, then brown, then they die.

Now, consider this carefully: it is the blood of the plant that gives life to the creatures that feed on it, and it is the light of the earth (sunlight) that is required to make chlorophyll.

Just as the blood of the plant (chlorophyll) is its life, the blood of man is also his life. This is well-documented, both in Scripture and by science. But let's take an even closer look at the design of the Creator.

How does man get his blood? A recent discovery gives a more complete answer than ever before. I am so excited to be able to share this knowledge with you!

The molecular structure of the basic unit of blood in the plant (chlorophyll) is almost the same as the molecular structure of the basic unit of blood of man (hemoglobin) except for the center atom. The center atom in the plant is magnesium and for hemoglobin it is iron.

Now listen to this: When man eats green plants, the blood molecule of the plant can become the blood molecule of man by a process biochemists could not describe until recently. It is called "porphyrin biosynthesis."

This, then, is the clincher of this unique story about blood. God in His marvelous wisdom provided perfectly for the self-repairing, self-rejuvenating, and self-energizing of the physical man through the blood of plants.

This makes chlorophyll a very important substance to you and me. If there were no chlorophyll, there would be no photosynthesis. If there were no photosynthesis, there would be no plant life. Without plants, there would be no animal life on earth, including us! Chlorophyll, therefore, is absolutely essential to life.

There is no substitute in nature for turnip greens, collard greens, mustard greens, beet tops, spinach, broccoli, kale, parsley, and other greens. They are chemo-protectors, chemo-preventors, chemo-attackers, chemo-reversers, chemo-alleviators, yes, chemo-healers. Green foods are the *real* chemo-therapists!

If you fail to eat green foods, you are failing to protect, prevent, reverse, or heal your body's cells. Is that what you want? Only you can decide.

2. Carotenoids: Orange and Yellow Foods

There is a "believe it or not" fact about these two colors; they are present wherever chlorophyll is present. The deep green color predominates, but the yellows and oranges are also present. Tomatoes are predominantly red, but the carotinoids (yellows and oranges) are also there, covered up by the red.

These colors are very stable; they are not easily destroyed by cooking. They are not very soluble in water and are not appreciably affected by acids or alkalies. They are closely related to vitamin A; our bodies can convert carotene into vitamin A.

3. Anthocyanins: Red Foods

Red, blue, purple — these foods are colored by red pigments called anthocyanins.

In the foods laboratory, it is fun to watch these foods during the cooking process. Red cabbage for example, can go from bright red through various shades of blue to green, depending upon how much acid (vinegar, lemon juice, etc.) is added.

There is not a wide variety of red foods. Berries of different kinds, plums, grapes, apple peeling, beets, eggplant, red cabbage, cherries, and red peppers are common anthocyanins. Still, they play an important health role — like everything created by God.

4. Flavones: White Foods

Practically all vegetables contain flavones, but they are covered over by the deeper pigments. Most flavones are solid white like cauliflower, but a few, like those in rutabagas, horseradish, parsnips, and yellow onion are cream-colored. Fresh ears of corn can be either color — white or yellow.

Let's look now at what these colors seem to achieve in our bodies when they are ingested.

Keep in mind that absolutely everything has been provided by nature to aid these self-healing, self-rejuvenating, self-energizing, self-renewing bodies of ours to:

- Fight off disease
- Slow down disease
- Reverse disease
- Heal disease: To build and rebuild cells, tissues, organs, systems (nervous, enzymatic, digestive, hormonal, structural, etc.) — *everything* — without much help at all from man and his manufactured concoctions.

Let's take a look at 16 of God's 23,000 or more medicines.

SIXTEEN DISEASE DESTROYERS

1. Sulforaphane
- Found in broccoli and cauliflower.
- Blocks the formation of tumors in mice even when they are excessively exposed to cancer-producing chemicals.
- Reverses tumors already formed.
- A recent article reports that broccoli sprouts contain up to 50 times higher levels of sulforaphane than the mature broccoli plant.
- A doctor from Johns Hopkins University, Dr. Talalay, reported that two pounds of broccoli a week can cut colon cancer risk by 50 percent.
- Good to reduce the risk of breast cancer also.

2. Isothiocynates
- Found in cabbage, watercress, turnips, Brussels sprouts, cauliflower, broccoli, mustard, and kale.
- Inhibit lung tumors caused by smoke.
- Heal stomach ulcers. (Two weeks of freshly squeezed cabbage juice can heal ulcers.)
- Stimulate anti-cancer enzymes.
- Block cancer-causing substances from reaching their targets.

3. *Curcumin*
- From the turmeric spice plant.
- Decreased tumors in tumor-prone animals from 41-91 percent.
- Helped rheumatoid arthritis patients.
- Patients had less morning stiffness.
- Decreased joint pain.
- Patients walked much easier.
- Lowers bad cholesterol quickly — within 48 hours.

So why not at least learn to like turmeric rice?

4. *Chlorophyll*
- Worldwide studies consistently ferret out dark-green leafy vegetables as perhaps the single greatest dietary discouragement to the development of certain cancers.
- Quickly heals bed sores.
- Improves skin texture — wrinkles.
- Detoxifies dietary poisons.
- Speeds healing of wounds by making "granulation tissue."
- Inhibits clumping of red blood cells.
- Is involved in healing a whole host of conditions, including deep surgical infections, fistulas, abscesses — almost any acute or chronic condition involving pus, and much more.
- Is anti-aging in many ways. (Read the whole chapter in my book *Green Leaves of Barley:*

Nature's Miracle Rejuvenator. There is a two-week period when young barley leaves contain a wide array of enzymes and nutrients that are not in the mature plant. (To order call 1-800-447-9772.)

5. *Carotenoids*
- Another phytochemical with lots of research behind them. They are the most colorful, economical, and widely available sources of carotene.
- Studies worldwide have linked carotenoid foods to a reduced risk of cancer — cancers of the esophagus, stomach, intestines, mouth, throat, bladder, and prostate.
- Carrots, pumpkin, sweet potatoes, winter squashes, and several yellow fruits are excellent sources of carotenoids.

6. *Genisteen*
- Found in soybeans and cabbage.
- Decreases prostate cancer.
- Decreases premenstrual syndrome.

7. *Capsaicin*
- Found in chili peppers.
- Decreases asthma and arthritis.

8. *Pectin*
- Found in fruits — apples are an excellent source.
- Decreases heart disease.

- Decreases cholesterol.
- Decreases high blood pressure.

9. *Anthocyanins*
- Produce the red color in blueberries, strawberries, red cabbage, grapes, all beans, beets, plums, etc.
- Decrease heart disease.
- Decrease cholesterol.
- Decrease high blood pressure.
- Nourish macular cells in the eye.

10. *Epigallocatechin Gallate (EGCGs)*
- Found in green tea leaves.
- Seal up tumor cells, preventing their growth or spreading. Dr. H. Fujiko of Japan was able to reduce the number of tumors by 73 percent in animals who had them by giving EGCGs from green tea leaves.
- Effective in deterring skin cancers, colon and stomach tumors, arthritis, poor circulation, allergies, asthma, lupus, and arteriosclerosis.

11. *Gingerol*
- From the ginger plant.
- Decreased inflammation in joints of arthritic patients.
- Does not cause stomach problems like aspirin-type painkillers.

- Soothes the stomach.
- Helps with airsickness and sea-sickness better than the drug Dramamine, according to research.

12. Lycopenes
- Found in tomatoes.
- Protect against lung and prostate tumors.

13. Allicin
- Found in garlic and onions.
- Decreases bad cholesterol by 42 percent.
- Breaks down blood clots and decreases high blood pressure.
- When you get both allicin and EGCGs, it's a double punch that can eliminate cholesterol from ever being a problem. (Three capsules a day of Bear Paw Garlic may rival all blood pressure drugs today, according to one doctor. To order, call 800-447-9772).

14. Flavonoids
- The white color in most fruits and vegetables.
- Deter heart disease.
- Destroy free radicals within arteries.

15. Quercetin
- A common flavonoid.
- Found to relieve common allergies.

- A study begun 25 years ago and finished in 1996 (McMaster University in Canada) had 12 medical schools in seven countries follow several thousand patients. Those who ate flavonoid foods had less illness from tumors and heart problems.

16. Ginkgo biloba
- Decreases artery blockage by 38 percent.
- Increases circulation and deters blood clots.
- Improves memory.
- Helps eliminate ringing within ears.
- Stops depression.
- Stops sexual impotency.
- Decreases retinal disease of the eyes.

These are only a few of the more than 20,000 known "destroyers" of our enemies.

THE TYRANNY OF TECHNOLOGY

A food science company says they hope to have 200 new foods on the market by the year 2000! Just what Americans need:

- 200 more abominations!
- 200 more dead foods!
- 200 more ways to make dead people!

Why are people in North America dying in epidemic numbers from heart disease, cancer, arthritis, diabetes, osteoporosis, liver and kidney failure, and all the rest? The answer is so simple that most people refuse to accept it. The truth is: Americans have accepted man's ideas instead of God's regarding food and other biblical disciplines for healthy living.

Let's look at what the "tyranny of technology" has accomplished:

- *Grains:* Decapitated, bleached, and robbed them of medicinal power.
- *Sugar:* Turned sugar beets and sugar cane into a narcotic, and we're all hooked!
- *Fat alternatives:* Produced man-made margarine and olestra — both unhealthy substitutes.
- *Meats* (chicken, beef, pork, etc.): Pumped animals full of drugs, hormones, and antibiotics, which adversely affect our health.
- *Milk:* Pasteurized, homogenized, and filled it with hormones.
- *Genetically altered foods:* Produced hybrid grains.
- *Designer foods:* Fabricated products like most ice creams, dairy creamers, and whipped toppings.
- *Microwaving:* Changed nature's structure of food.

What is the result of all these chemically-altered foods:

- *65-80 percent of our foods are not natural.*
- *65-80 percent of us are chronically ill.*

Don't forget, nutrition is not everything. It is the most important building block in the foundation for health along with exercise, clean water and air, sleep, rest, and hormones from happy thoughts.

All of these are a part of God's weapons for good health. God never intended for mankind to destroy himself with "fake" foods, or pollute the earth and water with poisonous waste, or sit around all day vegetating in front of a television.

It is my hope that every reader will begin to take Genesis 1:29 much more seriously. I want to see Americans reverse their diseases. God has already provided everything we need if we will only follow His plan.

WHAT IS BARLEYGREEN™?

BarleyGreen is a food concentrate (a powder) produced from the juice of young barley leaves and containing a wealth of nutrients: vitamins, minerals, live enzymes, chlorophyll, proteins, and other nutrients. This potent concentrate is blended with powdered brown rice, which is a rich source of vitamin B1, B2, nicotinic acid, and linoleic acid. BarleyGreen is also available with or without kelp.

1. What does BarleyGreen do?

Since BarleyGreen is a high quality, balanced, natural green food product, it helps the body balance, cleanse, and heal itself. A healthy body repels disease and enables one to enjoy life to its utmost.

2. Why barley?

After 13 years of intensive research on over 400 green plants, Dr. Yoshihide Hagiwara, a noted researcher, found that the young barley leaf was an extremely rich source of a broad spectrum of nutrients needed by the human body.

3. Is BarleyGreen safe for everyone to take?

BarleyGreen is grown entirely free from pesticides, chemicals, or preservatives. It has been used in Japan by over two million people for over 20 years, and in the U.S. for over 15 years without ill effects. Yes, it is safe.

4. How do you take BarleyGreen?

Start with one level teaspoon (or less) dissolved in a glass of cold water, juice, soy or rice milk once a day in the morning before breakfast. (Do not use hot liquids since the heat will deactivate the enzymes and other nutrients).

After a few days to a week, you may increase the serving to a heaping teaspoon once or twice a day, or even two to three teaspoons per day if you like. Chronically ill people have benefited from higher doses (ten or more teaspoons per day).

Because BarleyGreen is absorbed directly into the mucous membrane of the mouth and digestive tract, ideal absorption will take place if it is ingested 1/2 hour before or two hours after a meal.

WHAT NUTRIENTS ARE IN BARLEYGREEN™?

1. Vitamins and Minerals
BarleyGreen contains a balance of many vitamins and minerals. Most notably, it has a high potassium content. Many people note a diuretic effect like that achieved with "water pills." This is frequently followed by a lowering of an elevated blood pressure. The body seems to get in perfect balance.

2. Enzymes
Probably thousands of live enzymes exist, and 300 are known to be found in BarleyGreen. These chemicals help to speed up the numerous chemical reactions that take place in our bodies every second of the day. BarleyGreen contains a high amount of the enzyme superoxide dismutase, which is excellent for the heart.

3. Superoxide Dismutase (SOD)
SOD protects the body's genetic material (DNA) from injury caused by free oxygen radicals. This

protective action probably helps retard aging and, theoretically, might retard the development of cancerous changes in the cells.

4. Chlorophyll
Deodorizes, detoxifies, and aids healing. It also appears to help control allergies, build the blood, and help in blood sugar conditions.

5. P4DI
Suppresses stomach and duodenal inflammation and pancreatitis. It also acts as an anti-inflammatory like the steroids (but without the harmful side effects of steroids) and thus helps with arthritis, tendinitis, and other inflammatory conditions. It also stimulates DNA repair.

6. Proteins.
In addition to having all of the 18 essential amino acids, BarleyGreen has been found to contain a glycoprotein, which helps to lower blood pressure.

7. Alkalinity
BarleyGreen helps to neutralize the acidity caused by eating excess meats, starches, and preserved foods.

WHAT DOES BARLEYGREEN™ DO?

Double-blind studies conducted at several universities here in the United States and Japan provide the following scientific evidence of benefits:

- Several skin diseases respond and are healed.
- Endurance is increased.
- Growth rate in young mice was enhanced.
- Anti-fatigue activity increased.
- Inhibits tumor growth.
- Serum cholesterol was lowered.
- Has a strong anti-inflammatory activity.
- Anti-ulcer activity has been well documented.
- Inhibits toxic aldehyde.
- Young barley leaves have pharmacological activity, including anti-allergic effects.
- One of the first effects to be reported by new users is increased energy.

STOP TAKING FOOD SUPPLEMENTS?

Not necessarily.

Although BarleyGreen contains an excellent balance of most of the vitamins and minerals, you may add certain nutrients to attain maximal supplementation.

Phone 1-800-447-9772 for more information about BarleyGreen™.

Part 2

The Evangelistic Potential of Fasting

CHAPTER FIVE

Fast for the Hungry

This chapter is dedicated to those readers who know in their hearts that God has a plan for improving their own health with fasting while, at the same time, increasing their ability to contribute more resources to end-time ministries — especially those that feed spiritually and physically hungry people around the world.

This concept is not a product of modern times. In the 1800s, Adam Clarke wrote in his commentary on Isaiah 58:7:

Deal thy bread to the hungry. But this thou canst not do, if thou eat it thyself. When a man fasts, suppose he does it through a religious motive, he should give the food of that day, from which he abstains, to the poor and hungry, who, in the course of providence, are called to sustain many involuntary fasts, besides suffering general privations. Woe to him who saves a day's victuals by his religious fast! He should either give them or their value in money to the poor.[12]

After more than 60 years of teaching and experience in the area of foods and nutrition, one thing I know for sure: the truth about nutrition is a hard message to hear and accept with the heart. It is difficult for us to exchange present-day poor eating habits for a more healthful dietary lifestyle. Why? Because our rich, fatty, sweet, spicy foods *taste* so good! Healthy foods in comparison often seem less tantalizing!

Fast for the Hungry ministry is designed to help people deny themselves unneeded calories for the purpose of saving food dollars which, then, can be channeled to support Great Commission programs and projects. A major secondary goal is to instruct people on how to improve their health through better nutrition. (See chapter four on pages 116-120 as a beginning teaching.)

Inherent also in this ministry is the concept of self-denial. It should be obvious to every American that self-denial does not fit into the present predominant philosophy of our society. Millions of us have espoused a very liberal view of life; we are encouraged from many sources to "do our own thing," "be our own person," "decide what we want and go get it."

Subjecting ourselves to a rigorous program of self-denial is unthinkable to many. This, of course, opposes the truth of God's Word. Jesus said, "If anyone desires to come after Me, let him deny himself, and take up his cross and follow Me" (Matthew 16:24 NKJV). Our "cross" could easily be making a change in our eating and drinking habits.

Those who are willing to follow Jesus in self-denial will choose the path of discipline through fasting. Why? Because this humbling act symbolizes the utter submission of our will to the will of God.

It is my belief that the time in history is ripe for a change in our beliefs and behavior — especially our behavior. It is time for Americans to humble themselves, fast and pray, seek His face, and turn from our independent, self-indulging ways. Were this to happen, I believe we would hear from heaven, have our sins forgiven, and see ourselves and our nation healed. This is the challenge presented by Fast for the Hungry ministry.

It is my prayer that millions of people, not only Americans, will participate in this challenge.

IT CAN BE DONE

This idea of fasting for the hungry was first conceived by the author in 1979, when a study was conducted to see if such a project could succeed.

These were the results: In four weeks, 25 persons denied themselves nearly 500,000 calories, lost an aggregate of 87 pounds, and saved $599.96! It worked!

See how easily money could be raised for feeding hungry people?

If 100, 1,000, 10,000, or 100,000 persons could be motivated to follow this idea, it would be a cinch (without anyone getting a pay raise) to bring millions of dollars into worthwhile projects in a short period of time — and we would improve our health in the process.

Consider these figures:

Number of Participants	Dollars Saved in Four Weeks	Projected @ 1997 Prices for One Year
25	$ 750	$ 39,000
100	$ 3,000	$ 156,000
500	$ 15,000	$ 780,000
1,000	$ 30,000	$ 1,560,000
10,000	$ 300,000	$ 15,600,000
50,000	$1,500,000	$ 78,000,000
100,000	$3,000,000	$156,000,000

WHAT'S IN IT FOR YOU?

The expected results of this project are exciting.

1. Improved health.
Thousands could experience weight loss — with improved energy and longevity. Overweight illnesses (heart disease, high blood pressure, diabetes, arthritis, cancer, etc.) could be more easily controlled — and even reversed.

2. Financial benefits would accrue:
- God rewards sacrificial giving. (See Isaiah 58:6-12.)
- Fewer medical bills.
- Less money spent on drugs.
- Fewer days of work missed because of ill health.

3. Miscellaneous benefits:
- Spiritual growth.
- More energy to do God's work.
- Improved personal self-esteem.
- Increased longevity.
- God will be pleased!

HOW TO FAST FOR THE HUNGRY

The Fast for the Hungry ministry can be adjusted to any audience:

- An individual or family
- A church-sponsored program
- A secular group project

The main emphasis will be to ask volunteers to make a commitment to a definite plan or schedule of self-denial of unneeded calories (fasting). With this as one of the major goals, our techniques include:

- Asking you to make a personal fasting commitment or self-denial project for a given period of time.
- Asking you to "self-stylize" your program to suit your food preferences and meal patterns. You decide "how much" and "for how long" you will fast. We offer suggestions on page 179.
- Asking you to select the specific Great Commission project you or your group would like to support. (Your pastor or ministry director may give suggestions.)
- Offering help through a team approach to ministry. (We offer a teaching video and printed materials with follow-up ministry by local volunteers.)
- You may purchase related nutrition materials to assist you in understanding the value of this project. (Phone 1-800-447-9772.)

- You will be given facts about world hunger contrasted with facts about over-consumption of food in America.
- Emphasis on gaining new knowledge of biblical nutrition will be encouraged. I suggest my easy-to-read nutrition book to use: *Life-Long Health*. (Order from 1-800-447-9772.)
- Audience participation through question and answer periods will be encouraged when possible.
- A new video explaining the details of this project will be available at minimum cost for each participant desiring a copy.
- Fast for the Hungry ministry can furnish a sample copy of the food-denial record card, which suggests dollar/cents costs of many foods. (You may calculate exact costs yourself, of course, if you prefer.) A sample commitment card can be found at the end of this chapter.

THE POWER OF MULTIPLIED EFFORT

"A three-fold cord is not quickly broken" (Ecclesiastes 4:12 NKJV).

Business owners use many different methods to bring success to their ventures. For example, there are sole proprietorships, partnerships, corporations, and so forth. A recent business phenomenon that is producing great results for multitudes is network marketing. Harvard School of Business sees this as the wave of the future.

Many Christians, I am told, do not believe in multilevel or network marketing. However, let me show you how this concept could be very successfully used to bring in thousands of dollars from sacrificed food (and other things) for sharing with the poor. I am recommending it as one method to be used in this project.

Suppose you want to get involved in Fast for the Hungry, but you feel that your savings from not eating would be small — not large enough to even count for much of anything. Take a look at what you could do to change that image!

If you asked two other people to join you in: (1) denying unneeded calories; (2) saving the money they would have spent; and (3) giving the money to worthwhile projects, you would have significantly increased savings.

Let's go one step further. If each of your two new partners recruited two friends to do the same thing — and each of those persons recruited just two additional persons — your group would now total 30 people.

Surely, 30 people working together as a unit, encouraging and cajoling one another, could make a significant contribution to this project.

The simple drawing below shows you my proposal.

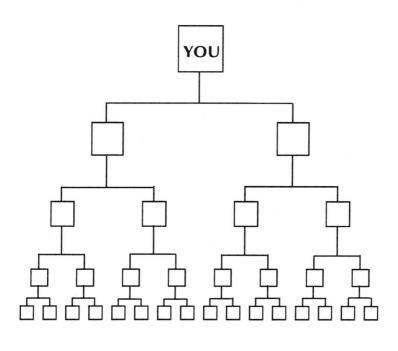

YOU + 2 + 4 + 8 + 16 = YOU + 30

(Concept taken from *Partners Magazine,*
American Image Marketing, Inc., Nampa, Idaho.
January 1995, page 15.)

Finding two individuals to cooperate with you in
this ministry should be easy to achieve for almost

everyone. Look what would happen if you found three persons to be in your group and, in return, each of them found two. You would have 45 people instead of 30 in your group.

The end result is that, rather than generating all the savings yourself, your efforts are greatly multiplied without any single individual doing a lot of work.

Networking your efforts for Fast for the Hungry will greatly increase your total savings. I hope you are challenged to give it a try and to become a demonstration of its power for humanitarian purposes.

Can such an endeavor be successful today? Absolutely! Your own "sacrifice" will be a good start.

OVERFED, UNDERFED — AND DYING

When we study the health statistics about the people of our world, two facts become painfully clear.

- Millions are overfed and dying prematurely because of it.
- Billions are underfed and dying tragically because of it.

1. Millions of people are overfed and dying.
Let's look at the facts.

- *One out of every four adults* in America is either overweight (10 percent or more above ideal weight) or obese (20 percent or more above it).
- An estimated 80 million overweight persons live in the United States alone! Of these, 34 million are thought to be obese.[13]
- Obesity contributes to 300,000 deaths a year in our country.
- Americans are the most overweight people in the industrial world.
- Being fat is no joke. It diminishes the quality of life, causes disease, and shortens life.
- Extensive research has linked being overweight with a whole host of devastating diseases. To name a few: cancer, diabetes, heart disease, osteoarthritis, cataracts, arthritis, gallstones, strokes, etc.

As Americans, we need to attack obesity with the same fervor we have used to educate people about the dangers of cigarette smoking.

2. Billions around the world are underfed and dying. Consider these tragic statistics:

- 1.5 billion persons lack adequate protein to live.
- An additional 1/2 billion are in the last stages of starvation.
- 40,000 people die *daily* from malnutrition.

This situation is difficult for us to comprehend since neither we nor our family and friends are among those numbers!

While I am sure God is saddened by the *unnecessary* deaths of His starving children, I am equally as sure that He is also saddened by the health statistics of His *overfed* children. Let's see what the statistics show.

CHRONIC ILLNESSES RELATED TO OBESITY

Here are some chronic conditions related to being overweight and/or obese when compared to adults of normal weight.[14]

- Cholesterol gallstones are 300 percent more frequent.
- Toxemia of pregnancy is 700 percent higher.
- Infection of urine-collecting part of kidney is 500 percent greater.
- Diabetes mellitus is 400 percent more common.
- There are more maternal deaths in childbirth.
- Infections are 200 percent more frequent.
- Post-operative mortality is 250 percent greater.
- High blood pressure is found 250 percent more often after age 45.
- Several types of cancer are more frequent.

- There is increased morbidity from digestive diseases.

Many other serious conditions such as gallstones, sleep apnea, osteoarthritis, and other disabling disorders of locomotion bear a direct relationship to obesity, although causality is not necessarily proven by these associations.

SPIRITUAL STARVATION

The world's imbalance in available natural food carries over into the spiritual realm.

- Two-thirds of the world lack adequate spiritual food: literature, Bibles, study materials, preach- and teaching to get people saved, filled with the Holy Spirit, and discipled.
- One-third of us are "choking to death" from over-possession and *over-consumption* of books, tapes, videos, Bibles of many translations, dozens of dictionaries, concordances, tracts, and many other tools. In addition, we enjoy Christian television 24 hours a day, plus conferences and seminars, study groups, teachers, preachers, evangelists, and prophets galore.

How can we help minimize this discrepancy?

EATING IS A SPIRITUAL MATTER

Are you glorifying God with your eating and drinking? If not, it is time to face the issue squarely.

To follow our own inclinations will not lead us to the right destination. Our sinful nature begs us to follow its desires which, incidentally, cause us to perish.

That idea comes directly from Scripture: "Therefore, brethren, we are debtors — not to the flesh, to live according to the flesh. For if you live according to the flesh, you will die; but if by the Spirit you put to death the deeds of the body, you will live" (Romans 8:12-13 NKJV).

The truth of this statement is substantiated by current statistics from life insurance studies of mortality.

Having scientific, nutritional knowledge is not, however, the whole story. The truth is: Eating is also a spiritual matter. It requires spiritual understanding and spiritual methods to control appetites and form good eating patterns. The Bible has a great deal to say about this problem.

SCRIPTURAL ADVICE ABOUT SHARING FOOD

Many verses of Scripture give specific directions for handling the problems of overeating and the hungry "brother-sister" issue. I have chosen to put these in the form of a true and false quiz. Take the test at the end of this chapter and tally your score to see where you stand.

What does the Bible teach us about our responsibility to the hungry and starving in this country and around the world?

- "'When you put on a dinner,' he [Jesus] said, 'don't invite friends, brothers, relatives, and rich neighbors! For they will return the invitation. Instead, invite the poor, the crippled, the lame, and the blind. Then at the resurrection of the godly, God will reward you for inviting those who can't repay you'" (Luke 14:12-14 TLB).

- "But if someone who is supposed to be a Christian has money enough to live well, and sees a brother in need, and won't help him — how can God's love be within him? Little children, let us stop just saying we love people; let us really love them, and show it by our actions" (1 John 3:17-18 TLB).

- "If you have a friend who is in need of food and clothing, and you say to him, 'Well, good-bye and God bless you; stay warm and eat hearty,' and then don't give him clothes or food, what good does that do?" (James 2:15-16 TLB).

- "This is the kind of fast I want . . . share your food with the hungry" (Isaiah 58:6-7 TLB).

SACRIFICE, SAVE, GIVE

The above verses answer two important questions:

- Do I have a responsibility to feed the hungry and help the poor?
- Will God hold me responsible for these acts?

The answer to both questions is a definite yes! Christians, especially, have a moral and spiritual responsibility for feeding the hungry and helping the poor.

As Americans we have developed food habits that are *not* in line with what science and experience have shown to be desirable. Our own survival depends upon our returning to the principles of good nutrition.

Christians are God's witnesses in the world, God's chosen people, His Bride for whom He is coming soon. Millions of us need to renew our vows of love for God and begin to live that love at the breakfast, luncheon, and dinner table. There we can continually *sacrifice* the eating of unneeded calories, *save* the money these calories would have cost, and *give* it to Great Commission programs and projects.

The Book of Proverbs tells us that if we will listen to God and obey His instructions, we will be given wisdom and good sense.

> Yes, if you want better insight and discernment, and are searching for them as you would for lost money or hidden treasure, then wisdom will be given you, and knowledge of God Himself; you will soon learn the importance of reverence for the Lord and of trusting Him (Proverbs 2:3-5 TLB).

What does God expect of us? His Word provides the answer: "Here is my final conclusion: fear God and obey his commandments, for this is the entire duty of man" (Ecclesiastes 12:13 TLB).

THE FOODS & NUTRITION "GLORY TEST"

Directions: Read the statements below. Circle the T if you believe and practice the thought expressed in each. Otherwise circle the F.

T F *I do everything, even my eating and drinking, to the glory of God (1 Corinthians 10:31).*
(One of my highest goals is to preserve my body so that God can use me for years of productive work.)

T F *God does not mean for me to eat more food than I need, so I don't (1 Corinthians 6:13).*
(I know I don't overeat because my weight is normal for my sex, height, age, and activity level.)

T F *I do not spend money on foodstuffs that don't do me any good (Isaiah 55:2-3).*
(I do not buy "empty calories" — foods in the form of sweets, soft drinks, alcohol, chips, candy, doughnuts, etc.)

T F *When I overeat, I soon get fat and bloated; then, in the midst of a plentiful supply of food, I forsake my God, as did the children of Israel (Deuteronomy 32:15).*

T F *The Bible says that honey is good for me, even in large quantities (Proverbs 25:16)*
(Oops! I had better read that verse again to make sure.)

T F *I regularly deny myself food by fasting as one way of humbling myself.*
(I know that those who humble themselves shall be exalted, according to Matthew 23:12.)

T F *I feel good about having my appetite under control now before Jesus returns for me.*

(Luke 21:34 lists "surfeiting" — excessive eating — as one of the important things we are not to be doing when Jesus returns.)

T F *I am a good example to others in my eating and drinking habits.*
(In all food matters, I am showing myself a pattern of good works, as commanded in Titus 2:7, John 13:15, 1 Peter 2:21.)

T F *I seldom stuff myself (although it all tastes good) because God's Word warns me against it (Proverbs 23:1).*
(Jesus said not to be overcharged with too full a stomach. I am obedient to Him because I love Him more than I love myself.)

T F *I do not want to be overweight or obese because if I defile or spoil my body, which is God's home, God will destroy me (1 Corinthians 3:16-17).*

Author's note: While there is not a valid way of scoring the above test, all statements are meant to be true except the one about honey, which is false.

How well did you do on the test? How well do you feel about your score?

Let's end this part of the test on a positive note. Proverbs 3:6 says, "In everything you do, put God first, and he will direct you and crown your efforts with success" (TLB). Keeping the laws of God will help you to have a long and happy life. (See Proverbs 4:4.) After all, isn't that the goal of every Christian?

THE TRUTH ABOUT WORLD HUNGER

You are now ready to take the next part of this quiz. These statements are designed to help us understand the implications of the worldwide problems of poverty and hunger.

Directions: Read the statements below. Circle the T if you think it is true, or F if it is false.

T F   *If I were someone whose annual income was $75 or less, I would not think my very, very rich neighbors should share with me.*
(An estimated one billion persons are in this poverty category.)

T F   *If all of my children and family members cried themselves to sleep every night because of the pains of hunger for food (which I have no way of providing), it would not disturb me.*
(At least 500 million parents face this problem daily.)

T F *Around 52 percent of the world's children under six years of age are victims of malnutrition.*
(True)

T F *I believe it would glorify God if we took care of our own citizens' food needs before leaving the shores of our country to feed people of other countries.*
(Regardless of your response to that statement, it is estimated that, in 1992, we have about 37 million citizens living below the poverty level in America. Who should take care of them? I believe the Church of Jesus Christ should; we could easily do that if every Christian tithed his or her income.)

THE TRUTH ABOUT OUR DIETARY EXCESSES

Directions: Circle your answer, T or F.

T F *If I am an average American, I routinely take in more calories than I need.*
(Most Americans eat an excess of around 300-400 calories daily.)

T F *Americans are eating three to four times more protein than our bodies need, especially too much red meat.*

(If I denied myself two 4 oz. servings of beef per week, that would release about 10-21 pounds of grain a week. In a year, that could serve about 2,080-4,160 persons one cup each!)

T F *By consuming an average of 130 pounds of sugars and sweeteners per person per year, Americans are increasing their risk of 59 "poor health" conditions.*
(Diseases known to be associated with high sugar consumption are: obesity, tooth and bone destruction, diabetes, cancer, heart disease, osteoporosis, etc.)

T F *Americans are consuming too high a percentage of calories from fatty foods.*
(Examples of foods high in fat, which could be advantageously decreased, are fatty meats, sausages, bologna, cream, margarine, fried foods, doughnuts, chips, ice cream, salad dressings, mayonnaise, shortenings, and oils.)

T F *Adults in the USA consume much more salt (sodium) than they need.*
(The major health hazard associated with an excess of sodium is high blood pressure.)

WHAT YOU CAN DO

You — and every American — can help alleviate the food consumption problems that exist between "the haves" and the "have nots" of our generation while improving your own health.

It has been estimated that Americans are around *two billion* pounds overweight. How many calories are required to produce this overweight condition? Around *eight trillion*. These are, of course, all *unneeded* calories. How much money did all these unneeded calories cost? *Billions* of dollars!

The calories required to maintain (nourish) two billion pounds of fat cost about $9,315,068 per day. This totals $3.4 billion in one year at 1997 food prices.

If we brought our weight to normal levels, we could save in food resources $8.1 billion in one year. (A one-time savings, of course.)

It takes about 574,000 gallons of gasoline *per day* to carry our excess fat around with us. At $1.30 per gallon, that costs about $746,200 per day or $275 million per year.

In 1996, it has been estimated that the price of obesity among the American people is $100 billion annually.[15] That figure is up from $5 billion annually in 1976! Where will we be in another 20 years if we don't control our eating?

As a Christian, I ask myself and I ask you two questions:

- How do you suppose God feels about this?
- What do you think He would have us *do* about it?

My own special calling is to ask Christians to *deny* themselves unneeded calories, *save* the money they would have cost, and *give* it to Great Commission programs and projects.

Since He asked me to do this, I am fully persuaded that He will speak to *your* heart as to ways that we, together, can accomplish His purposes.

Yes, Christian friends, *eating is a spiritual matter.*

"Recite my laws no longer and stop claiming my promises, for you have refused my discipline, disregarding my laws" (Psalm 50:16 TLB).

What do we say to our millions of physically and spiritually hungry neighbors and families?

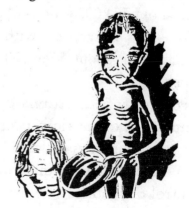

GOD'S REWARDS FOR OBEDIENCE

Isaiah 58:6-7   Proverbs 22:9
2 Corinthians 9:9   Galatians 2:10
Proverbs 14:31

- "I want you to share your food with the hungry."
- "To help the poor is to honor God."
- "He who gives to the poor shall never lack."
- "He that pitieth the poor lendeth to the Lord and He will pay him again."

If we implement God's ideas about feeding the hungry, what rewards if any, can we expect to receive? In other words, what's in it for me?

Excellent rewards always follow when we are obedient to God's ways. The paternal aspect of God the Father is no more clearly seen than in this principle: Obedience to God is always rewarded.

Here are a few of the verses that tell us what to expect if we share our food with the poor or hungry:

- Proverbs 28:27: "Your needs will be supplied" (TLB). (But a curse will be upon those who close their eyes to poverty.)
- Psalm 112:9: "Your deeds will never be forgotten; you shall have influence and honor" (TLB).

- 2 Corinthians 9:7-9: "Your own needs shall be met and you'll have plenty left over to give joyfully to others" (TLB).
- Proverbs 22:9: "You will be a happy man" (TLB).
- Proverbs 19:17: "You will be lending to the Lord and he pays wonderful interest on your loan" (TLB).
- Luke 6:35: "You shall be called the children of the highest" (KJV).
- Psalm 37:26: "Your seed will be blessed" (KJV).

These commands and promises from God's Word lead us to four conclusions:

- We are to share.
- It honors God.
- Sharing brings blessings to us.
- God repays us for helping the poor.

Isaiah 58:5-12 (TLB) lists many rewards from obeying this command: "If you fast the Lord's fast, feed the hungry and provide for the poor, then:

- God will shed His own glorious light upon you.
- He will heal you.
- Your godliness will lead you forward, and goodness will be a shield before you.
- The glory of the Lord will protect you from behind.

- When you call, the Lord will answer, "Yes, I am here." He will quickly reply.
- Your light will shine out from darkness, and the darkness around you shall be as bright as day.
- The Lord will guide you continually and satisfy you with all good things, and keep you healthy too.
- You will be like a well-watered garden — like an everlasting spring.
- Your sons will rebuild the long-deserted ruins of your cities, and you will be known as "The People Who Rebuild Their Walls and Cities."

WHAT IS THE LORD TELLING YOU?

"And this is the secret: that Christ in your hearts is your only hope of glory" (Colossians 1:27 TLB).

If Christ is in *your* heart, what would He have you do in regard to denying yourself, saving the money, and giving more to feeding the physically and spiritually hungry?

"The Lord of Hosts says, 'Get on with the job and finish it! You have been listening long enough!'" (Zechariah 8:9 TLB).

MY COMMITMENT

Having felt in my heart that there are calories or other commodities or services that I could deny myself for use in Great Commission projects or programs in these last days, I hereby commit myself for the following pledge:

Items to be Denied	*Number of Weeks*	*Cash Value*
_____		
_____		
_____		
_____		

Total Denial
Commitment $_____

- Drink pure water as your only beverage for one day / one week / one month.

- Sacrifice all desserts and "sweets" for one day / one week / one month.

- Sacrifice one meat serving per day for one week / one month.

- Fast one meal a day for one week / one month. Preferably not breakfast.

- Fast one day a week.

- Substitute a salad lunch for a regular lunch.

- Save "snack food" money for one week / one month.

- Eat "home-cooked" meals for one week instead of "restaurant meals."

- Come up with your own ideas for saving your Fast for the Hungry money.

APPENDIX A

Certified Fasting Physicians & Clinics

For a list of certified fasting physicians and their clinics, send a self-addressed, stamped envelope to:

Mark Huberman, Secretary/Treasurer
International Association of Hygienic Physicians
4620 Euclid Boulevard
Youngstown, OH 44512

Phone: 330-788-0526
Fax: 330-788-0093

APPENDIX B

Fasting Helps

Here are suggestions for some appropriate liquids to drink while fasting. Rotate the recipes to add variety.

1. Take 1 teaspoon of BarleyGreen in juice or water after arising in the morning. You may have up to 10 teaspoons a day, if needed, to keep your body happy.

(For more information about BarleyGreen™, phone 1-800-447-9772.)

2. Make a drink from the following ingredients and have a glass every hour or two:

1 gallon distilled water
1 1/2 cup fresh lemon juice (cleanser for liver and kidneys)

1/2 cup maple syrup (real)
1/4 teaspoon cayenne pepper (opens up blood vessels)

3. Make a broth from vegetables (any you like) such as:
- Cabbage
- Potatoes
- Onions
- Tomatoes
- Turnips
- Carrots
- Green beans
- Celery and celery leaves
- Crook-neck squash
- Zucchini
- Bragg Liquid Aminos to taste

Chop any combination of vegetables and cover them with a large amount of water (three quarts of water to each quart of veggies). Cook covered for 30 minutes. Turn off the heat and let veggies stand in water.

Your family can eat the veggies; you drink only the broth. One or two quarts per day will boost your energy level.

4. Drink freshly squeezed vegetable juices. Carrot — or carrot and apple — are excellent. Carrot and BarleyGreen or parsley is also quite fulfilling.

5. Dr. Julio Ruibal considers a juice made from 1/3 carrot juice, 1/3 celery juice, and 1/3 green leaves juice to

be an excellent fasting drink. (1 teaspoon of BarleyGreen can be substituted for the green leaves.)

6. Drink 64 oz. of pure water or other liquid beverages per day on your fast. Add fresh lemon juice to some of your water. This helps normalize pH.

7. Drink herb teas. Have all you want, hot or cold.

8. Drink fruit juices — fresh, frozen, or canned. Dilute with 1/3 pure water. Limit your intake because of high sugar content.

9. I like homemade onion soup broth — just don't eat the onions.

10. Some people drink ginger ale. I find it to be quite sweet. A few sips won't hurt you.

Also:

- Take time to pray.
- Keep praising God for everything you can think of!
- Relax.
- Listen to beautiful music.

ENDNOTES

1. *Webster's New World Dictionary*, 493. (See bibliography.)
2. Derek Prince, *Shaping History Through Prayer and Fasting*, 7. (See bibliography.)
3. Bill Bright, *The Coming Revival*, 23. (See bibliography.)
4. Finis Jennings Dake, *Dake's Annotated Reference Bible, The Holy Bible*, 724. (See bibliography.)
5. Dick Eastman, *Love On Its Knees: Make a Difference by Praying for Others*, 77-81. (See bibliography.)
6. *Webster's New World Dictionary*, 657.
7. *Webster's*, op. cit., 22.
8. Derek Prince, op. cit., 85.
9. Dr. Julio Ruibal, *Fasting: Spiritual Weapon, Physiological Wonder*. (See bibliography.)
10. Paul C. & Patricia Bragg, *The Miracles of Fasting*, 82. (See bibliography.)
11. Adam Clarke, *The Holy Bible with Commentary and Critical Notes, Vol. III*, 766. (See bibliography.)
12. Adam Clarke, op. cit., *Vol. IV*, 217.
13. Theodore B. Van Itallic, M.D. and Artemis Simipoulous, M.D., *Obesity*, chapter 1, p. 1.

14. E. A. Lew, L. Garfunkel, "Variations in Mortality by Weight Among 750,000 Men and Women," *Journal of Chronic Diseases* 32:563-576, (1979).

15. *Barron's,* July 1, 1996, 25.

BIBLIOGRAPHY

Bieler, Henry, M.D., *Food Is Your Best Medicine* (New York, NY: Random House, 1965).

Bueno, Lee, *Fast Your Way to Health* (Springdale, PA: Whitaker House Publishers, 1991).

Bragg, Paul C. and Patricia, *The Miracle of Fasting* (Health Science, Box 7, Santa Barbara, CA 93102).

Bright, Bill, *The Coming Revival* (New Life Publications, 100 Sunport Lane, Orlando, FL 32809, 1995).

Clarke, Adam, *The Holy Bible with Commentary and Critical Notes* (Nashville, TN and New York, NY: Abingdon-Kokesbury Press, 1826.)

Dake, Finis Jennings, *Dake's Annotated Reference Bible, The Holy Bible* (Dake Bible Sales, Inc., P. O. Box 1050, Lawrenceville, GA 30246, 1981).

Eastman, Dick, *Love On Its Knees: Make a Difference by Praying for Others.* (Every Home for Christ, P. O. Box 35950, Colorado Springs, CO 80935).

Fuhrman, Joel, M.D., *Fasting and Eating for Health* (New York: St. Martin's Press, 1995).

Kirban, Salem, *How to Keep Healthy and Happy by Fasting* (Harvest House Publishers, 17895 Sky Park Circle, Irvine, CA 92707, 1976).

Medical Training Institute of America, *Basic Care Bulletin #4*, "How To Discover The Rewards Of Fasting" (Oak Brook, IL, 1992).

Prince, Derek, *Shaping History Through Prayer and Fasting* (Derek Prince Ministries International, P. O. Box 19501, Charlotte, NC 28219, 1973).

Prince, Derek, Booklet: *Restoration Through Fasting*, 1970.

Ruibal, Dr. Julio, *Fasting: Spiritual Weapon, Physiological Wonder* and video tape: "Fasting" (Julio Ruibal Foundation, P. O. Box 1830, Pinellas Park, FL 33780-1830, 1995).

Shelton, Herbert M., *Fasting Can Save Your Life* (Chicago, IL: Natural Hygiene Press, 1973, 122-124). (Dr. Shelton has fasted over 30,000 persons.)

Smith, J. Harold, *Fast Your Way To Health* (Nashville, TN and New York, NY: Thomas Nelson Publishers, 1979, 29).

Wallis, Arthur, *God's Chosen Fast* (Ft. Washington, PA: Christian Literature Crusade, 1968).

Webster's New World Dictionary, Third College Edition (New York, NY: Simon & Schuster, Inc., 1988).

INDEX

PRODUCT LIST

Resources Available from Swope Enterprises

BOOKS BY DR. MARY RUTH SWOPE	PRICE
Green Leaves of Barley: Nature's Miracle Rejuvenator (Updated Edition, New '96) Other translations available	$ 9.95
Surviving the 20th Century Diet: Scientific Solutions to a Diet Gone Wrong (New '96 — The Abridged Version of *Green Leaves of Barley*)	$ 6.95
Some Gold Nuggets in Nutrition (Enlarged and Updated for '96)	$ 4.00
The Roots and Fruits of Fasting (New '98)	$ 9.95
The Spiritual Roots of Barley	$ 5.00
Lifelong Health	$ 7.95

Listening Prayer	$ 5.00
Fasting . . . Spiritual & Physical Benefits	$ 1.00
Bless Your Children Every Day	$ 9.95

OTHER RECOMMENDED BOOKS

What Your Doctor May Not Tell You About Menopause by John R. Lee, M.D.	$13.00
Green Barley Essence by Dr. Yoshihide Hagiwara (Abridged version available)	$10.95
Health in the 21st Century by Francisco Contreras, M.D.	$18.00
God's Way to Ultimate Health by Rev. George H. Malkmus	$18.95
Why Christians Get Sick by Rev. George H. Malkmus	$ 8.95
Recipes for Life from God's Garden by Rhonda J. Malkmus	$24.95
Country Life Vegetarian Cookbook edited by Diana J. Fleming	$ 9.95
Ten Talents Cookbook by Frank J. Hurd, D.C., M.D. and Rosalie Hurd, B.S.	$21.95
Antioxidants, Coenzyme Q10, Ginkgo Biloba by Dr. E. S. Wagner, Ph.D. (each $1.00) or "Trio"	$ 2.95
Fasting and Eating for Health by Joel Fuhrman, M.D.	$24.95
Cleansing the Body & The Colon by Teresa Schumacher and Toni S. Lund	$ 3.95

Of These Ye May Eat Freely by Jeani McKeever	$ 3.95

AUDIO CASSETTE TAPES BY DR. SWOPE

Newer Concepts in Nutrition (New in '98) Two-tape set	$ 8.00
The New Health Model (New in '98) Two-tape set	$ 8.00
Use Blessings Everyday (Single tape)	$ 3.00
Understanding the Family of Plants and Research: *The Foundation Stone* (New in '96)	$ 4.00

VIDEO TAPES

Nutrition Update . . . BarleyGreen by Swope/Darbro (30 min.)	$16.00
What to Eat & What Not to Eat by Dr. Swope (60 min.)	$20.00
It's Not Too Late: Nutrition Update by Swope/McKeever (58 min.)	$20.00
Using Nutrition as Medicine by Swope/McKeever (43 min.)	$20.00
You Can't Improve on God! by Lorraine Day, M.D. (77 min.)	$21.00
Cancer Doesn't Scare Me Anymore by Lorraine Day, M.D. (77 min.)	$20.00

NOTICE TO INTERNATIONAL ORDERS:
ALL PRICES ARE IN U.S. FUNDS

All Prices Subject to Change Without Prior Notice

SHIPPING & HANDLING

$ AMOUNT	U.S.	CAN	INT'L
$0 and up	$ 3	$ 6	Call
$10 and up	$ 4	$ 8	Call
$20 and up	$ 5	$10	Call
$30 and up	$ 6	$12	Call
$40 and up	$ 7	$14	Call
$50 and up	$ 8	$16	Call
$75 and up	$ 9	$18	Call
$100	$11	Call	Call
Over $100			
Repeat Chgs			
Case GLB	$15	Call	Call
Case BYC	$15	Call	Call

To place an order, please contact:

Swope Enterprises
P. O. Box 1290
Lone Star, TX 75668

1-800-447-9772
or
903-562-1504
Fax: 903-562-1609